The Daily Telegraph

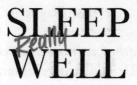

SLEEP
Really
WELL

The Daily Telegraph

SLEEP
Really WELL

DR PAUL CALDWELL

ROBINSON
London

Constable & Robinson Ltd
3 The Lanchesters
162 Fulham Palace Road
London W6 9ER
www.constablerobinson.com

First published in Canada by Key Porter Books Limited, 2001

First published in the UK by Robinson,
an imprint of Constable & Robinson Ltd, 2003

Adapted for the UK by Dr Ian Smith

A copy of the British Library Cataloguing in Publication Data
is available from the British Library.

Publisher's Note: This book is not intended to be a substitute for medical
advice or treatment. Any person with a condition requiring medical
attention should consult a qualified medical practitioner
or suitable therapist.

ISBN 1-84119-672-X

Printed and bound in the EU

10 9 8 7 6 5 4 3 2 1

Contents

Acknowledgements

As a family physician, I spend a large part of my day-to-day contact with patients making science understandable to them – their symptoms, diseases, and treatments. In this book I am indebted to the scientists of sleep who have, through their experiments and observations, made an understanding of the complexity of sleep possible. Many prominent Canadian and American sleep physicians working in sleep laboratories across the continent have provided the scientific information that is the basis for this book. In addition, Dr B. Squires realized how important it is to transmit accurate medical information to the public. It was he who arranged for the partnership with Key Porter Books.

I would also like to thank Anna Porter of Key Porter Books, for giving me the chance to write this book, and Renée Dykeman, for helping me with the editing process.

Thanks also are due to Susan DeLong, for typing the manuscript and for her patience and support.

Last, I would like to thank my eldest daughter, Jen, who helped me overcome writer's block.

Dr J. P. Caldwell, CCFP(C)

Foreword

Sleep is one of life's great mysteries, whose inner secrets have defied legions of scientific investigators over the past five decades. To be sure, its several stages – five in all, from the 'twilight zone' downwards – have been described with great clarity; the physical effects of chronic sleep deprivation have been itemized; sleep related disorders and their consequences have been elaborated. But the fundamental question of what initiates and maintains sleep and the source of its extraordinary restorative powers remains elusive. The best that can be said, as Paul Caldwell points out, is that sleep is 'as complicated a physiological state as wakefulness'.

From a practical perspective, most people's main interest in sleep is to get enough of it, and of the right sort – restful and refreshing. When this is not obtainable, for whatever reason, they naturally wish to know what to do about it. These are significant matters, as the extensive correspondence that follows every mention of sleep in my weekly column in *The Daily Telegraph* confirms. Problems such as insomnia, night waking and the perplexing sleep-related syndromes are almost universal.

At least in future I will be able to commend this lucid book confident that whatever the problem may be, readers will find it sympathetically dealt with.

Dr Caldwell challenges the common belief that sleep problems, especially as one gets older, simply have to be lived with. Rather, as he makes clear, it is surprising how many are readily preventable. Thus a brief list of the most important physical symptoms that disrupt sleep will include night cramps – avoidable by a glass of tonic water or quinine sulphate tablets at night; the foul sensation of restless legs syndrome – eliminated by low doses of anti-Parkinson drugs; heartburn – abolished by acid-suppressant drugs and placing a couple of telephone directories under the head of the bedstead; the exhausting ritual of night waking to pass large amounts of urine – preventable by the drug Desmopressin that 'resets' the normal biological rhythm production. And so on.

Similarly, the chronic sleep deprivation caused by insomnia does not 'have to be lived with'. As Dr Caldwell shows in a whole chapter devoted to this issue, there is almost a superfluity of possible alternative remedies to the standard sleeping pills. The best-known stems from the clever realization that the drowsiness induced by the older type of antihistamines – used for the treatment of hayfever and other allergic conditions – could be turned to therapeutic advantage as a simple hypnotic with minimal side effects. But there is now also a long list of natural remedies, readily available from the local health food store, to choose from including Valerian, especially popular in Europe, camomile tea, lemon balm, Verbena and others.

Finally, no account of sleep would be complete without some reflections on that most inscrutable of brain phenomena, the nocturnal 'movie in the mind' – dreaming. 'Dreams have the remarkable ability to solve the problems of the day,' Dr

Caldwell observes, 'so artists dream about art, plumbers about plumbing, musicians about music' – and their dreams can be a major source of creative inspiration. Thus the novelist Robert Louis Stevenson could dream complete stories in a single night, and return to them night after night to change their endings. Or again, the Italian composer Giuseppe Tartini named one of his more haunting melodies, the famous *Devil's Trill Sonata*, because he first heard it in a dream – being played by the devil himself on a violin!

Sleep Really Well is a most useful – and entertaining – guide to a fascinating subject. I commend it highly.

Dr James Le Fanu

Introduction

For each of us, every single day of our lives, the need for sleep is a powerful biological force. Every twenty-four hours or so, we simply must lie down and rest for a period of time or we will be unable to continue to function. This regular requirement for sleep is so pressing, so demanding that, though it may be delayed or deferred, sleep cannot be denied completely. We all spend one-third of our lives asleep; it is simply part of the human condition, a basic requirement of life. In the pages that follow, this phenomenon of human sleep is explored as a natural history we all share.

Until the 1950s sleep was thought to be a single night-long blankness of thought, not even worthy of studying, but the discovery of rapid eye movement or dream sleep suggested that perhaps there was more to it than first appeared. We now know that sleep is as complicated a physiological state as wakefulness, and the recent advances in understanding of the biology of sleep will be immediately applicable to your own pattern of rest.

Poor sleep limits the ability to function and to enjoy life, and the whole discipline of sleep medicine has evolved to study the reasons why this basic human need for rest is not adequately met in so many people.

I believe that sleep is very important to us all and that solid refreshing sleep can make a tremendous difference in the quality of your life, allowing you a joy and peace denied to those who sleep poorly. This book will, I hope, give you the knowledge to once again sleep like a baby, and awake refreshed and renewed every morning for the rest of your life.

1

Where Were You When the Lights Went Out?

Imagine that it's a few minutes after 10:30 p.m. and you have just finished watching the evening news. You're relaxed and content, slouched down in your most comfortable chair. When the sports scores flash across the television screen, you flick the picture off and, as is your habit, you begin the process of going to bed. You lock the doors, check the children in their rooms and, satisfied that all is well, slip off your clothes, put on looser garments, brush your teeth, and slide wearily into bed.

Warm and secure, you reach over and turn off the bed-side light.

The day is over; you're ready for sleep.

Closing your eyes, you lie there expectantly, knowing that soon sleep will wash over you. For several hours, you will be swept away by sleep into a world where time has no meaning. If you are lucky, you will awaken, after what seems to be just a few seconds, to see the sunshine of a new morning. You will feel refreshed and renewed, your mind clear and your body revitalized – literally a daily rebirth.

But have you actually ever considered what happens when you close your eyes and sleep? Have you ever wondered about the process that snatches away all those hours between bedtime and morning, when the alarm rings and you regain control over your mind and body? The nature of sleep has intrigued scientists for years, but only recently have they explored and understood the particulars of this fascinating other world.

The Conditions of Sleep

Let's follow you through a typical night's sleep.

When you lie down to sleep in the evening, you've already established, by your routine, several necessary conditions for you to be able to go to sleep. You've checked the security of your house, protecting yourself from danger. You've opened the bedroom window for fresh air and adjusted the covers so you are just the right temperature. You've bunched up the pillow so your head is neither too high nor too low. You've read for a while (nothing too spicy) so your mind can ease away from the stimulations of the day, and, of course, you've turned out the light, decreasing the sensory input to your resting brain.

These conditions are very important for the process of initiating sleep. Many people find it impossible to go to sleep until certain requirements, which vary from person to person, are met. Once these conditions are met, you lie quietly in bed anticipating sleep.

What Is Sleep?

It's fairly difficult to define sleep precisely, but an acceptable definition is that sleep occurs when one is no longer aware of the external environment. Lying in bed, you are still well aware of the ticking of the clock or the breeze rustling the leaves outside the window, or, perhaps, even the quiet of the room – you're simply resting; you're not yet asleep.

The time it takes to go from this resting state to sleep varies tremendously, but it's often short – about fifteen minutes. Most believe that falling asleep is gradual, but entering sleep is sudden, often taking just a few seconds. In an interesting experiment, several subjects had their eyelids taped open and a bright strobe light flashed before them every second. The subjects were instructed to press a small button after each flash to confirm that they had seen it. For ten or fifteen minutes they regularly tapped their responses to the flashing light. Suddenly, they stopped – they had fallen asleep in an instant. When awakened at that time (yes, it is possible to fall asleep with your eyes taped open), they reported that they did not remember having missed any flashing lights at all! What happened? Within a second or two, they went from being awake to being asleep.

THE TWILIGHT ZONE
When you are truly asleep, you are not responsive to the outside world. Sleep researchers have identified five different patterns, or stages, of sleep and you have just entered the first one, which I call 'the twilight zone'.

There was a television programme that once began: 'You're travelling through another dimension – a dimension not only of sight and sound but mind; a journey into a wondrous land whose boundaries are that of imagination.' This is what scientists refer to as the first stage of sleep. Sleep researchers can identify exactly when experimental subjects 'fall' asleep – when they leave the world of the awake behind them.

THE ELECTRICITY OF SLEEP

The human brain is like a huge, continuously operating computer, and the amount of electricity generated by the brain can be measured. With a sensitive enough instrument, this electrical activity can be detected by sensors or electrodes as far away from the brain as the scalp, employing exactly the same principle used to check the function of the heart with an electrocardiogram (literally, a picture of electricity of the heart). If these same electrodes or sensors are placed in various areas on the scalp, they can pick up the electricity produced inside the brain. This measurement is called an electroencephalogram (EEG). The word has the same beginning as 'electricity', plus the Greek word for brain, *encephalon*, plus *grapho*, to write. It is literally the writing out of the electrical pattern of the brain.

When the EEG was first used, scientists found that the best electrode was a small pin stuck into the scalp of the patient. Nowadays EEGs are painless – the electrodes are simply taped to strategic spots on the scalp. EEGs are used to record the electrical activity in all sorts of conditions, such as epilepsy, but when the measurement technique is used on sleeping patients, remarkable changes in electrical patterns are seen.

As befits the biological computer that it is, the human brain produces different patterns of electrical activity when it's awake or asleep. Obviously, when the brain is sleeping, some electrical activity persists – you still breathe, your heart still beats, you may have dreams, etc., and all these functions require some electrical activity. When doctors first began doing EEGs on sleeping patients, they believed they would find a single pattern characteristic of the sleep state, different from that present in the waking state, and it would be consistent throughout the whole period of sleep.

Surprisingly, they found not one but five different patterns, five different states of activity of the brain, and each pattern was associated with a different type or depth of sleep. These they called the 'stages of sleep'.

THE FIRST FEW MINUTES OF SLEEP

When you've entered what I have just called 'the twilight zone', you've entered Stage I sleep. Your EEG tracing is different from one taken when you were awake, and you are no longer completely aware of your external environment. A fairly soft noise may awaken you – perhaps a whisper, or a light touch – but you're much less responsive to the environment than you were just a few minutes earlier when you were awake. The electrical activity in your brain is different.

Often, at this early stage in sleep, you are aware of slow, rambling, disconnected thoughts, and you may feel as if you are falling or floating. You feel quite relaxed; your muscles lose their tenseness, and a feeling of peace, ease and pleasure envelops you. This is the stage of relaxation reached in yoga meditation. Your eyes roll lazily beneath their closed lids; the muscles of your body begin to slacken; your breathing becomes regular and predictable; and, in about ten minutes, you enter the second stage of sleep.

This second stage is much like the first, except it has its own EEG pattern, reflecting another change in the electrical output of the brain. Stages I and II are both transitional stages, literally 'twilight zones', because they are transporting you from the awake state to the deeper sleep stages that follow. In Stage II sleep, it takes a stronger sensory stimulus – a louder noise, a greater change in temperature, or a heavier touch, for example – to bring you back to the awake state. Sometimes during these early twilight-zone stages of sleep, you may experience a sudden jerk – your arms and legs suddenly contract forcefully and you quickly wake up out of sleep, startled. If you have observed this phenomenon in your bed partner you know it's quite dramatic – a sudden jerk in bed, and then he or she is completely awake. This occurrence is perfectly normal and of no great significance, though the phenomenon is poorly understood. At any rate, the twilight zone of sleep – Stages I and II – lasts about thirty minutes, so that half an hour after you went to bed, you're entering the next stage: deep sleep.

THE SLEEP OF BABIES

Deep sleep is as good as it gets – 'sleeping like a baby' – and if falling asleep is like descending in a lift, deep sleep is the basement level. Deep sleep (Stages III and IV) is a truly restful and fulfilling experience. It's wonderful. As you lie in bed in deep sleep, there is little body movement; your heart rate and blood pressure both fall and become stable, and the electrical activity in your brain shows a slowing of regular activity. You are, in fact, more or less dead to the external environment – 'more or less' because you still can be awakened, even though a much stronger stimulus is necessary to bring you round. Whereas in twilight-zone sleep you could be awakened with a soft whisper, it now takes the ring of the telephone or the smoke alarm, since you are that much farther away from the external world. Your muscles are deeply relaxed, your eyes hardly move, and you are as far distant from the awake state as you ever are in sleep.

Have you ever been at a party with children where, as the evening wears on, they eventually cannot resist the drowsiness of the late hour, no matter how hard they try? Inevitably, they fall asleep wherever they are – on the sofa, in your arms, on the floor, and so on. When you yourself become tired and decide to leave, you lift the children up to take them to their bedrooms or to your car to take them home. The children act as if they are in a comical kind of coma. They don't wake up when you lift them; they may speak in drowsy, garbled language, but they do not resist your attempts to move them – they simply hang on as you carry them, quickly moving to a comfortable position wherever you put them, and then going back to sleep. Next morning, they don't recall the episode at all. This is the wonder of deep sleep.

If you are aroused from deep sleep, you won't find yourself wide awake and thinking accurately, but rather confused and slow to react. It seems to take a long time to rise from the basement level of sleep back to the ground level of normal thought processing.

We still don't really know why we sleep, but this deep, or Stage III or IV, sleep is thought to be the most restorative part of the sleep experience. During deep sleep the levels of growth hormone rise. This hormone not only promotes growth in children, but also repairs and rebuilds in adults. This type of sleep is thought to be necessary for the restoration of both physical and mental capability.

This deep-sleep restorative phase lasts about twenty to forty minutes, and then you begin to rise again towards the awake state, entering twilight-zone sleep, and then a curious thing happens – you wake up!

Awakenings Common

Well, you don't actually wake right up, but you come quite close to the awake state. You rise in level from deep sleep up through Stage II, and then through Stage I, towards the awake state. You become aware of your environment once more; in fact, you usually alter it. You turn over, bunch up your pillow to get it just right, pull the covers up to chin level, and then, often in only a couple of minutes, descend again through the stages of twilight-zone sleep back to the deeper levels of drowsiness.

This 'partial awakening', as it's called, is an important event to understand. We don't simply stay in deep sleep all night long. Scientists reason that, for an evolving species such as *Homo sapiens*, it was important to be able to check the security of the sleeping environment regularly while obtaining the benefits of rest. We are quite vulnerable in sleep, particularly in deep sleep, and these partial awakenings are thought to function to help protect us.

We shift position by moving around in the bed, and this action prevents pressure sores from developing on our skin. Medical patients who, for some reason, such as drug overdose, are prevented from moving while 'asleep' develop skin ulcers from the weight of the body pushing down and forcing blood from areas of the skin in contact with the bed; when the skin is deprived of nourishment, it quickly dies and large sores result. We avoid this kind of pressure phenomenon every night by moving regularly during sleep.

We also check the room in which we sleep, and are sensitive to changes in temperature, noises, smell, and, of course, changes in lighting. In short, all our senses are employed in a rapid evaluation of the environment in which we sleep. Satisfied that all is well, you close your eyes and begin the descent again. Very quickly, you descend through the twilight zones and, in fifteen minutes, enter the next phase of sleep – by far the most exciting.

REM SLEEP: A DIFFERENT KIND OF SLEEP
Up to this point, you have been asleep in the classic meaning of the word – that is, your brain has been dozing and only a few of the basic circuits were working. Your body also has

been resting. Though you did move around, your body has been on autopilot, without specific instructions from the sleeping brain. Now, however, all that is about to change – you're in for the midway-ride excitement of rapid eye movement (REM) sleep, where the brain wakes up.

In *Miss Saigon*, the musical, one of the Vietnamese prostitutes sings about 'the movie in my mind' – her dream of a better life. With REM sleep, you're about to star in your own home movie, on your own big screen, with quadraphonic sound, in your own bed, and in your own mind. Not only will you star in it, but you will also be the only one in the audience. Rapid-eye-movement sleep is the ultimate in home entertainment.

REM sleep is a fairly new discovery. In the 1950s, sleep researchers began to notice the rapid flitting motion of the eyeballs beneath the closed lids in sleeping subjects. The sudden jerky motion was easily observed behind the closed eyelids, and the eye movement was identical to that exhibited when the subject was awake and watching some activity in real life. Curious about what was happening to the sleepers when their eyes began to move rapidly around, researchers woke the sleeping subjects up as soon as the movement was noted. Almost 85 per cent of those so awakened said they were dreaming, and they could relate the details of the dream readily. The motions of the eyes in REM sleep are widely believed to be the result of the sleeper 'watching' the events in the dream. Researchers concluded this by measuring the movements and correlating them with the dream content. For example, watching a tennis match produces a characteristic back-and-forth, horizontal movement of the eyes. It seems that the sleeping eyes are following the activity in the dream just as they would in real life – but with one important difference.

When we're awake, the eyes see various patterns of light and dark, and these impulses are sent to a part of the brain, the occipital cortex, to be registered as objects and activities. We 'see' through our eyes. In sleep, the opposite appears to happen – it seems that the dream (the thing we 'see') originates in the brain, and the eyes move back and forth while watching it play. You're actually 'seeing' with your brain and following with your eyes something your brain is imagining!

At the same time as they noted the eye movements, sleep researchers noted a different pattern on the EEG – a pattern very similar to that produced when the brain is wide awake. The sleepers themselves were very still, exhibiting little or no movements (except those roving eyes), but the electrical activity of the brain was almost the same as when the brain was wide awake. This combination of increased brain activity and markedly decreased activity of peripheral muscles is characteristic of REM sleep.

When you enter your first REM sleep, your brain goes into high gear, but if we looked in at you in your bed, we would see no movement except for your breathing and your eyes darting around beneath closed lids. A profound paralysis of the muscles of your body is seen in REM sleep, and your arms and legs lie motionless. What is happening is that the impulses from your very active brain are blocked high in the spinal cord, preventing you from moving any of the large muscles of your body. Because the nerves to your eyes arise from the brain at a higher level than the spinal cord, they are unaffected by this blockade.

In REM sleep, the block of transmission of impulses is chemical rather than mechanical. You are essentially paralyzed, just as you would be if your neck had been broken. The paralysis of the body is temporary, and easily reversed when you awaken, but otherwise it is the same.

If you think about it, you'll see that this is good planning: it prevents you from acting out the dreams your brain is enjoying. You may twitch a bit in the face or legs, perhaps whimper or make a garbled sound, but in general you're unable to respond to any of the acts in the dream, except to watch.

We've all had the opportunity to observe the paralysis of REM sleep whenever the family dog enters this phase in his snooze. (Yes, animals have REM sleep too.) When the dog begins to dream of unimaginable canine delights, he may make little whelping sounds; perhaps a paw will begin to tremble, and his nose to twitch; and, if you look closely, his eyes will be darting back and forth beneath their lids, following the sights and sounds of his own movie.

FIELDS OF DREAMS

If we were to awaken you after a few minutes of REM sleep, you could probably tell us the particulars of the dream. It's true that some people 'dream' in twilight zone or deep sleep but these dreams seem to consist most commonly of a single scene or feeling, whereas in REM sleep everyone dreams with the frenzied action and movement of a Hollywood feature attraction. We all dream every night (as long as we enter REM sleep), though we rarely remember these dreams in the morning. Dreams often involve some degree of frustration at being unable to move. This is of course because you are unable to move – the activity of the dream is witnessed by your sleeping brain without any possibility of your muscles responding to the action. This often accounts for the particulars of the dream, your inability to affect the course of events of the dream. We've all had this feeling. You may, for example, in the dream be in the situation where you are being chased by a gruesome, bloodied murderer and yet are

The Sleep of Animals

Almost all mammals sleep – with the same kind of EEG changes and sleep stages and architecture as humans. The tiny mouse and the huge elephant, the monkey and the bat, all have very similar alternating patterns of deep and REM sleep, and similar patterns of sleep behaviour. Some animals sleep for much of the time – the giant sloth and many bats sleep up to twenty hours a day, but the giraffe sleeps only two hours a day and the horse only three. Many adult mammals have the same percentage of REM sleep as humans do – about 20 to 25 per cent, but the percentage of REM sleep, and indeed sometimes the amount of sleep, depends on whether the animal is a predator or prey species. It seems that safety and protection are important prerequisites for adequate sleep, and for REM sleep. Animals that are prey species, such as most herbivores (cows, sheep, goats, etc.), sleep fitfully – they don't have much REM sleep and their amount of sleep in general is a much smaller percentage of the twenty-four-hour day than those animals that are predators (such as the big cats, which sleep up to 70 per cent of the time). The common ground squirrel, a prey species, is able to achieve a deep sleep of fourteen hours a day by living in an extensive burrow, safe and sound. On the other hand, a rabbit, which lives in the tall grass and nests on the surface or occasionally in shallow burrows, is only able to sleep two or three hours at a time and usually achieves only up to 10 per cent of REM sleep.

Surely the most interesting sleep of all animals studied is that of the black sea dolphin, an aquatic mammal. Like most sea-living mammals, the dolphin sleeps at the water's surface, with its blowhole just breaking the waves, but the impressive thing about this creature is that it is able to allow only one hemisphere of its brain to go to sleep at a time. Literally, half of the dolphin's brain will be in deep sleep for an extended period of time – two to four hours on average – while the other half of the brain is wide awake. After this time, the hemispheres reverse! It seems that the dolphin has evolved this method of sleeping to protect itself (by keeping half of its brain awake and so maintaining some alertness).

Thus the sleeping pattern of humans can be identified as part of a development of sleeping patterns in the rest of the animal species of the earth.

powerless to strike out against him or even to escape. This paralysis, in spite of intense mental activity, has a biological basis.

Accompanying the dreams of REM sleep, the pulse rate rises and falls with the action, as does the rate of breathing and the blood pressure. This increase in blood pressure and pulse is thought to be one of the main reasons why heart attacks and strokes are common at night. When we're asleep, the heart and blood vessels should be at rest – but they're not. Instead, they are responding to the emotional effects of the dreams we all have, and since blood flow to the brain is increased four times during REM sleep, this is a time of increased risk.

PENILE ERECTIONS DURING REM SLEEP

Curiously, blood flow to the genital organs is also increased, in both sexes. This causes penile erections in men and clitoral engorgement in women. In the male, these erections during REM sleep occur even in infants inside the uterus, and they continue in most men until age sixty or seventy. The erections, which are usually full, begin about the time that REM sleep begins, and they last the entire length of the segment of REM sleep. This means a healthy adult male will have an erection that will last for twenty to thirty minutes at a time. The erections occur with most REM periods, regardless of the content of the dream, even dreams that are not remotely of a sexual nature. Because we usually have three to four episodes of REM sleep per night, that means in men an erection is present 20 to 25 per cent of the total time asleep. The purpose or function of such genital congestion during sleep is not known – it may simply be the result of paralysis of the peripheral nerves at the spinal cord, allowing the intrinsic nervous tissue of these organs to act in an unopposed fashion, freed from the inhibitions of the sleeping brain.

OTHER CHARACTERISTICS OF REM SLEEP

Several other things are interesting about REM sleep. First, you don't often snore. Snoring occurs more frequently in deep sleep, and it's caused by vibration of the soft palate and the uvula, the long flap of tissue that hangs down the back of your throat. Second, temperature regulation ceases during REM sleep. You don't perspire if you are hot, or shiver if you are cold. When you wake from a dream, you might be dripping perspiration from emotional reaction, but during the dream itself you are unable to change your temperature by either sweating or shivering.

Throughout REM sleep the brain behaves as though it is already 'awake'. It's hard to distinguish the EEG of REM sleep from the awake state, and, indeed, if you are awakened, your mind is quickly oriented and functions well, displaying none of the confusion or fog of deep sleep.

This whole state of REM sleep is so unusual that many sleep researchers have suggested that we in fact have three different states of consciousness – the awake state, the sleep state (by which they mean the deep-sleep state), and the state of being half awake (the brain) and half asleep (the body), or REM sleep.

THE STAGES OF SLEEP

Stage		Light transitional		
Stages II	}	or 'twilight-zone' sleep	}	Non-rapid-eye-
Stage III	}	Deep restorative		movement sleep
Stage IV	}	sleep		
REM		Rapid-eye-movement or dream sleep		

The Rest of the Night

You've just finished your first REM sleep of the night, though it won't be your last. You enter the twilight zone again, steadily rising towards your second partial awakening of the night. You check the room again, turn over to the other side, adjust your pillow, and return to sleep. You have just completed what sleep researchers call the first 'sleep cycle' of the night – that is, the whole pattern of sleep we have just described from when you went to bed until now. A sleep cycle begins with descent into twilight-zone sleep, then deep sleep, then rises again to twilight zone, and finally enters REM sleep. This cycle usually lasts about ninety to one hundred minutes, and most adults have three to five such cycles per night of sleep. Deep sleep predominates in the early evening's rest, but REM sleep dominates in the early morning; this explains why, when you awaken with the alarm clock, you are quickly oriented and able to function. Because the last cycle of the night often ends with REM sleep, you may awake with some memory of a dream.

Why do we have this alternating pattern of REM sleep with deep sleep? The answer is not known and is unlikely to be simple. Most researchers agree that deep sleep is restorative – it allows the body and mind to rebuild and recharge their respective batteries. Deep sleep is necessary for the well-being and physical health of the organism, and your body insists on it. If you've missed sleep your next sleep period will consist of a greatly increased amount of deep sleep, with very little REM sleep, as if your system demands this stage of sleep for renewal.

REM sleep, on the other hand, is thought to be necessary to allow the brain to sort information and emotion while the physical body rests. The analogy is drawn with a computer that needs to sort out its files and reclassify information regularly, though this and other theories are unproven.

Morning Has Broken

It's morning and the alarm has just gone off. You open your eyes to sunlight and vault out of bed with well-rested muscles and a clear mind, ready to take on the world. Over the night, you've spent about 25 per cent of your time in deep sleep, the same amount in REM sleep, and about half the night in twilight-zone sleeps and partial awakenings. It's interesting that quadriplegics (who have no muscle movement, and therefore no need to 'rest' their muscles) need just

---

Why Do We Yawn?

If you ever happen to have the privilege of observing a newborn baby, just minutes into this bright new world, you will notice that, in addition to belligerent crying, and stretching out of both arms and legs, yawning is one of the earliest movements of these tiny creatures. It's also present in many other animals – it has been observed in all classes of vertebrates, in birds and in reptiles and even in some fish. However, in spite of its wide distribution in the animal kingdom, no one seems to know exactly why we yawn.

Basically, yawning is a physical phenomenon that reflects a mental state of decreased arousal or boredom. The physical action of yawning is much the same as the physical action of smiling, grinning or crying. These are all physical movements that come about as a result of a mental or emotional state. They do not have a purpose other than to reflect that mental state in a social manner, with a physical sign that is easily recognized by others of the species. If you are happy, you smile – and that smile is a social communication to others of your mental state. If you are sad, you cry, and your tears are an easily visible sign of your emotional turmoil. If you are bored, weary or apathetic, you yawn. The wide opening of your mouth and inrush of air has no specific physiological function – it doesn't 'do' anything, but it signals your mental state to those around you, just as the smile or the laugh does.

as much sleep as everyone else. But people who are made to lie immobile in bed all night long with their eyes open and are not allowed to sleep do not feel refreshed in the morning. It seems we need this combination of physical rest and mental rest to achieve the benefit of sleep.

How Much Is Enough?

How much sleep is enough depends very much on the person. The requirements vary dramatically from person to person.

Salvador Dali, the surrealist painter, felt that he didn't want to waste a lot of his life sleeping, so he stopped sleeping in the usual sense, preferring a series of short naps each day. He would nap in a comfortable chair, holding in his hand a set of keys over a metal plate on the floor. When he fell asleep, the keys would fall from his hand onto the plate, and the noise would awaken him. He felt this short period of rest was enough to rejuvenate him.

Dali was an exception. The average adult sleeps between seven and seven and a half hours per night. Some 20 per cent of adults sleep less than six hours and 10 per cent more than nine hours per night. Generally, you need enough sleep to be able to wake easily, maintain alert wakefulness during the day, and yet be able to fall asleep the next night without difficulty. Don't fight it. Some people need more sleep than others, just as some need larger shoes than others. The art is figuring out how much sleep you need and making sure that you get it.

2
Time for Sleep

We as a species have a daily need for sleep. In any twenty-four-hour period, as a general rule, most of our time is spent awake and the rest sleeping. This daily pattern of alternating wakefulness and sleep is called the 'sleep–wake cycle' or 'rhythm'. It's an inherent biological programme tied to time – an internal periodicity or clock – and is very important for the understanding of sleep difficulties.

We don't stay awake for days on end; and we don't sleep for days on end either. We normally have some sleep and some wakefulness dividing up each twenty-four-hour time period, and the sleep–wake clock does the dividing. It says, 'It's time to go to bed. You feel tired,' and later, 'It's time to wake up; you feel refreshed.' Day after day, year after year, this need to spend part of the time sleeping makes itself evident.

This alternating rhythm of sleeping and being awake is only one of many such cycles or rhythms in the human body. For example, the secretion of cortisol, the hormone of stress, follows a basic daily pattern as well. It rises in the early hours of the morning and reaches a peak at about 7:00 a.m., then gradually falls to a low point about midnight. The secretion of this hormone from the adrenal gland occurs in this pattern not once a week or once a month, but every single day.

Similarly, the secretion of growth hormone reaches a daily peak during the early hours of sleep, then falls during the remainder of sleep and stays low for the rest of the day. The secretion of acid in the stomach reaches a peak between 10:00 p.m. and 2:00 a.m., and body temperature varies from a low at about 3:00 a.m. to a high at about 7:00 p.m. All these cycles have their own peaks and troughs, which recur predictably and daily.

Cycles or rhythms such as these that occur about once every twenty-four hours are called 'circadian rhythms' (from Latin *circa*, meaning about, and *dies*, meaning day). There are other rhythms in the human body that occur over a much longer cycle than twenty-four hours – the menstrual cycle is an example – and many biological rhythms occur over a much shorter period – such as respiration. However, the circadian rhythms of the sleep–wake cycle, temperature variation, and hormone secretion are very important for adequate sleep.

Refreshing sleep is possible only when all these multiple cycles are operating in harmony.

Internal Clocks, External Clocks

Though each and every one of us sleeps almost every day, the time we go to bed and the time we awake are only rarely dictated by our own individual need for sleep, by our own internal clock. Most of us go to bed not only when we are tired but also when the external world says it is time – that is, when the late-night news is over or when the hall clock

Sleep in the Menstrual Cycle

Sleep is different in women than it is in men. Between the ages of twenty and forty, women tend to go to bed earlier than men, usually take longer to fall asleep than men, and sleep for a longer period of time. More women than men complain about poor sleep – almost twice as many, and this seems to vary with the menstrual cycle.

In general, the best sleep occurs early in the menstrual cycle, just after the period, when oestrogen levels are slowly rising.

The difficulty with sleep seems to come in the premenstrual phase, a week or so before the period, and often persists into the period itself. During this time, tiredness and lethargy are common. Awakenings increase, and the amount of deep sleep is much less. Unpleasant dreams are common, and excessive tiredness can be seen, perhaps due to increased levels of progesterone (which has been shown to have a sedative effect).

The changes in sleep with the menstrual cycle are very individual – and many studies show little change in sleep at all. Premenstrual changes in sleep are commonly associated with other symptoms of the pre-menstrual syndrome such as weight gain, fluid retention, breast engorgement and mood changes. Treatment of the premenstrual syndrome itself often improves the quality of sleep in such patients.

reads 11:30. We are directed by some clock other than our own internal one. Can you imagine going to bed whenever you felt tired, without so much as glancing at your wristwatch? Most often the clocks in our lives play a very important part in our bedtimes; we even say, 'It's time for bed', as if somehow the time measurement were the priority, not the feeling of fatigue.

Similarly, it's the rare adult who is able to sleep as long as he or she wants. Our bedside alarm clock dictates the length of our rest. Of course, we have to get up to go to work, or to school, or to some other activity; sleeping in our modern society is structured by external demands on our time.

What would it be like if we could simply go to bed whenever we felt sleepy, awake when we felt refreshed, and then sleep again whenever we felt tired? Would our pattern of sleep be significantly different? Would we sleep for longer periods? Would the process of sleep be the same for humans released from the pressures of time and schedules, from electric lights and alarm clocks, and from all the other external reasons to sleep and wake?

If we accept that *Homo sapiens* has evolved from an earlier hominid, has our sleep evolved as well? What would the pure, unobstructed sleep of humans be like?

THE SLEEP OF CAVEMEN

Questions such as these were answered in 1938 by two early pioneers in sleep research, Nathaniel Kleitman and Bruce Richardson. They wanted to see what would happen to the natural rhythm of sleeping and waking in an experiment where there were no clocks, no external clues as to time – no schedules, no set mealtimes, no artificial reasons to sleep or to wake. They decided that there should also be no exposure to sun, because the cycle of dark and light is a kind of clock itself. They volunteered themselves for a month-long experiment. However, they had one major problem: they couldn't find an ideal location. Every building they chose had windows to the outside, or doors that let in the sounds that were signals of morning or evening, or other times in the external world. They finally settled on a most appropriate laboratory setting to examine the sleep patterns of primitive man – a cave! They chose Mammoth Cave in Kentucky, a huge subterranean labyrinth of rooms and halls and passageways. It was perfect – for thirty-three days they lived in the damp cave with a constant temperature of 54°F (12°C), without any idea what time it was above. This pioneer work, as well as several other experiments in various caves around the world, began to show what humans' 'pure' sleep was like.

In all these experiments, people released from the day-to-day time cues of dawn and dusk, of meal schedules and time restraints, chose their own pattern of sleeping and waking, directed by their own internal clocks. They still maintained part of the twenty-four-hour day awake and part asleep, but there was a very important difference between their sleep–wake cycle and the sleep–wake cycle of the people outside the caves. This important difference is a biological quirk that is responsible for much of the difficulty with sleep in our modern world.

The cavemen–scientists tended to go to sleep each 'day' about one hour later than the day before. Thus, at the end of a week, they were going to bed seven hours later than the people above them in the external world. Though they didn't know it, the cavemen–scientists were actually going to bed at dawn.

This finding is important because it means that the free-flowing sleep–wake cycle – unhindered by external cues such as sunlight and alarm clocks – repeats itself about once every twenty-five or even twenty-six hours, not twenty-four hours.

Those outside the caves geared their sleep to a twenty-four-hour schedule. They knew, for example, that their office opened every weekday at 9:00 a.m. and they were expected to be there. Their supper was usually on the table at about 6:00 in the evening, and the nightly news was over by 11:15, and so on. The cavemen were different: their 'day' was actually twenty-five or twenty-six hours long. Instead of being awake for sixteen hours and then sleeping for eight hours (the pattern of everyone outside the cave), the scientists inside the cave stayed awake for seventeen hours, then slept for eight hours.

The important concept here is that the natural human tendency is to have a sleep–wake cycle longer than twenty-four hours – a tendency that is out of phase with the real world.

Our internal timing doesn't fit that of our external world. The basic unit of time on earth is the daily turning of the planet away from the sun, a twenty-four-hour phenomenon.

With a natural sleep–wake cycle longer than twenty-four hours, we must somehow reset our timing every single day, adjusting our internal clock to match the external clock tied to the rotation of the earth. Otherwise we, like the scientists in Mammoth Cave, would soon be out of phase with the sunlight. To understand how we reset our timing each day it is necessary to examine the internal clock itself.

Sleep researchers have been able to isolate the exact spot in the brain where the internal sleep–wake clock resides. If you put your finger on your forehead just above your nose, between your eyes, the 'clock' lies about 2 inches (5 centimetres) in, a pea-sized bit of brain tissue that dictates when you feel sleepy. The clock sits on top of a bundle of nerve fibres that originate in the retinae of the eyes – the nerves that actually do the seeing at the back of your eyes. These nerves from both eyes cross and intermingle in this area, and this suggested to scientists that visual images, especially those of light, may have an effect on the clock, a fact that enabled them to explain the paradox of the conflicting time schedules. The criss-crossing fibres of the retina that form the base of the internal clock hold the clue to how we daily reset our clocks. Light – specifically, bright sunlight – is now known to be the most powerful influence on the sleep–wake system. Other influences affect it each day, such as hunger and mealtimes, social times (such as the beginning of school or the whistle to end a shift at work), regular wake-up time and regular physical activity (such as walking to work), but none is as important as light. That's one reason why blind people have trouble sleeping; they miss this most powerful regulating force.

All these time-setters, or time cues, are called *Zeitgebers* (from the German *Zeit*, meaning time, and *Geber*, meaning giver) and they are the external influences that reset our own internal rhythm to the twenty-four-hour day. Consistent *Zeitgebers* mean our sleep–wake cycle is appropriate for the earth's rotation. Failure to pay attention to time cues such as daylight allows our sleep–wake cycle to revert to its own intrinsic pattern, and we are soon sleeping inappropriately. In shift work, irregular sleeping schedules, jet-lag syndrome, and many other sleep difficulties, inconsistent *Zeitgebers* or time cues are the problem.

SLEEP–WAKE CYCLES IN THE VERY YOUNG AND VERY OLD

As any mother knows, newborns have no specific sleep–wake cycle; they simply sleep irregularly around the clock. At age six months or so, they establish a fairly predictable pattern of sleeping between thirteen and fourteen hours out of the twenty-four, and usually most of this time is at night.

Young children, until the teenage years, are usually the ones who have the least problem sleeping. Their circadian sleep–wake cycle is almost exactly twenty-four hours. They have no trouble going to bed and awakening at the same time each day; they seem to be the most efficient sleepers. When they become teenagers, however, their sleep–wake rhythm lengthens. It's usually closer to twenty-six hours for this age group. That means, for example, that if teenagers were to participate in the experiment in the cave, they would go to bed *two* hours later each night. Anyone who lives with teenagers recognizes that trying to get them to bed at a reasonable hour is difficult. There is a biological reason for this; regardless of what the hall clock may say, their own internal clock says they're not tired yet.

When they finally do go upstairs to their 'caves', they go to sleep but find it difficult to wake up at 8:00 the next morning.

The problem is worse on weekends, because their biological rhythm is even more at odds with that of the external world. On Fridays and Saturdays, because school is out for the weekend and they are free from the confines of studying and rising at a particular time, they are allowed to stay up later and sleep in longer. They go to bed an hour or so later on Friday night and sleep in an hour or so later than usual on Saturday morning (they're only following their own intrinsic rhythm). On Saturday night they go to bed another hour later (now two hours out of cycle) and sleep in two hours on Sunday morning, oblivious to the bright sunlight outside.

Sunday night, when they realize they must get up and go to school the next morning, they try to go to bed at the usual time, but of course they're two hours out of phase and find it difficult to go to sleep. The next morning, Monday, they are awakened by that pesky alarm clock only three-quarters of the way through their usual restorative sleep. It's simply a case of not resetting their internal clock carefully each day.

By contrast, for many elderly people the circadian sleep–wake rhythm shortens to significantly less than twenty-four hours. That's why Grandfather goes to bed at 7:30, just an hour and a half after supper. His biological clock tells him it's time for sleep. The same clock tells him to awake early the next morning, to begin the new day. His internal rhythm, being shorter than twenty-four hours, needs to be reset each day as well – by the same *Zeitgebers* the teenager responds to.

Failure to understand the importance of this basic biological pattern often results in inefficient sleep.

UP WITH THE BIRDS: LARKS VS. OWLS

As is true of most human characteristics, there is considerable variation in sleep–wake cycles. We all need to sleep for about a third of the twenty-four-hour day, but we differ in our own natural inclination to sleep. This difference is exemplified by two extremes: those whose peak alertness occurs in the mornings and those whose peak alertness occurs later in the day. These two opposites are extreme examples of the individuality of our sleep–wake cycles.

If you are one of those people who enjoy early rising, feeling refreshed and alert soon after awakening, chances are you are a morning person, or lark. The meadowlark, after which this pattern is named, is a popular songbird whose cheerful sound greets the rising sun with enthusiasm – the birds are active even before dawn. The bird is a symbol of industry and joy, and so are the human 'larks' – cheerful and enthusiastic in the morning, their performance best at this time. Larks generally are good sleepers, and are able to wake early without alarm clocks. They tend to fade as the day wears on, and to avoid late nights, preferring early to bed and early to rise. Their pattern of sleeping and waking has been accepted as laudable by modern society, and they are seen as industrious, punctual and efficient. They are 'normal workers', ideally suited for a nine-to-five job.

If you find that it takes a long time for you to reach your peak in the day, you're probably an owl, or evening person. Owls are, of course, nocturnal birds, and all their activity takes place during the night. They spend their days sheltered from the sun, in some protected spot, and if disturbed during the day they are dopey and sluggish. Human 'owls' share these characteristics – they have difficulty rising in the morning and often take a long time, sometimes hours after getting out of bed, to feel fully wide awake. They are not at their performance peak in the mornings, but usually come to life later in the day, often in the late afternoon or evening. They prefer to retire much later in the twenty-four-hour day than larks do, often after midnight. They sleep the same amount of time as anyone else – and, in fact, their sleep architecture is normal – but their peak alertness occurs later in the day. As a result, they have difficulty with regular nine-to-five jobs; they are simply not at their best until halfway through the working day.

Their sleep–wake cycle, delayed as it is, is viewed by society as less acceptable than the larks' – owls are often seen as lazy or unreliable instead of simply out of shift. Their performance, though just as valuable as the larks', tends to peak later in the day, so they often end up taking irregular or evening jobs, allowing them to be their best at work.

Both of these types are extremes. Most of us fall somewhere between these two patterns. By identifying your own type, you can understand your own strengths and weaknesses.

Circadian Peaks and Troughs: The Siesta Phenomenon

It's 1:30 in the afternoon somewhere in rural Spain. The sun is directly overhead and beats down with a bright heat that cannot be avoided. Somewhere, out of sight, a dog barks lazily. It's the midway point in the day, halfway between dawn and dusk, but the streets lie deserted. Even the village square is empty, except for a few perspiring tourists. The shops are all closed and abandoned. It's siesta time, and throughout the village, on beds and sofas and hammocks and chairs and benches, the Spanish are enjoying a brief midday nap. Soon they will return to their activities and responsibilities refreshed and relaxed.

Siestas are very much a part of the culture of Spain and

Latin America, but they are also observed in many parts of Africa and Asia. They are in fact an example of yet another circadian rhythm – the cycle of rising and falling levels of alertness, or wakefulness, throughout the day. Just as our temperature changes throughout the day, and hormone secretion varies from time to time, we tend to be sleepier at certain times of day than at others, and more alert at some times than at others, even if we are well rested.

Usually, the period of greatest alertness occurs in mid-morning, from 9:00 to 11:00, and there is a second peak of increased alertness in the early evening, between 7:00 and 9:00. Many people feel at their best in these hours of the day, and their energy and performance are maximal at these times. In experiments, subjects were brought into the sleep laboratory every single hour and asked to try to go to sleep. Most of them found it very difficult, if not impossible, to fall asleep at these times of increased alertness.

In contrast, the time of lowest alertness occurs between 3:00 and 5:00 a.m., with a second trough in midafternoon. At these times, subjects in the sleep laboratory fall asleep very easily. Most people who have been up an entire night will recognize this pattern; you will feel most tired in the small hours, between 3:00 and 5:00 a.m., then seem to get a 'second wind' in the early morning.

It's important to emphasize that these variations in the urge for sleep are present even in well-rested subjects; in sleep-deprived subjects, the tendency to fall asleep at 3:00 a.m. may very well be overpowering.

The Spanish siesta occurs at the beginning of the afternoon dip in alertness – the midday meal, the tropical heat, and the acceptance of this social custom combine to permit a short, restorative nap. The siesta cultures reduce their night-time sleep, so the total sleep over twenty-four hours remains on average eight hours. Many industrialized societies frown on afternoon naps but curiously encourage coffee breaks to maintain vigilance, using caffeine to counter the inherent decreased alertness.

Catastrophes and Circadian Troughs

We tend to be born at night, and to die at night. Spontaneous labour and birth are most likely to occur between 12:00 and 6:00 a.m., and a major peak of deaths occurs between 4:00 and 6:00 a.m., with a second smaller peak between 2:00 and 4:00 p.m. Heart attacks occur most commonly between 6:00 and 10:00 a.m., and strokes are most common between 5:00 and 6:00 a.m. These peaks are all associated with the period of greatest sleepiness, between 3:00 and 5:00 a.m.

Because these hours of greatest sleepiness are the hours of poorest performance, when alertness and vigilance are at their lowest level, it's not surprising that the greatest number of single-vehicle accidents (i.e., driving off the road) occur between 2:00 and 6:00 a.m., with a second peak between 1:00 and 4:00 p.m.

In a similar vein, dozens of studies have shown that industrial accidents, often caused by poor performance and decreased alertness, are more likely to occur during the two circadian troughs. There is no question about it: the times of increased sleepiness are significant risk factors for injury and disease, and these tendencies are aggravated by prior sleep loss.

Shift Work

At age forty, Peter had it made. He had everything society worships – a fulfilling job, a beautiful home, financial freedom, and, best of all, a caring wife and two wonderful young sons who adored him. To add to his good fortune, he had just been given yet another promotion at work – this time to the position of supervisor of the night shift.

There was no doubt about it – Peter was a winner. So why was this dynamo, this champion, sitting weeping in my office?

He looked old and tired, and he was crying openly. Some men cry silently – their tears, like their pain, simply welling up from inside and flowing out. Peter wept with loud abandon, catching his breath in huge, wet gasps.

'I think I'm losing it!' he cried. 'Sometimes I get so mad I could hit someone, and other times I just don't give a damn.' He squeezed the damp wad of tissue in his fist. 'Why don't they just leave me alone?'

What was it that took the joy from this man's life? What was the problem that made this pillar of strength a blubbering baby? It was simply the chronic sleep deprivation caused by shift work.

ORIGINS OF SHIFT WORK

Though it has caused immeasurable suffering, shift work is a very recent invention. Throughout thousands of years of evolution, human beings were less active, and certainly less productive, at night. We had no choice – the dark was simply too overpowering; we rested and slept in the poor light, marrying our natural need for sleep to the regular turning of the earth away from the sun. This made sense because we were much more vulnerable in the dark, and our survival was so dependent on sight that we were threatened when the natural sources of light were absent.

We were then, and are now, diurnal animals.

But Thomas Edison, the American inventor, changed all

that when he sent the newly found power he called 'electricity' through a fine wire in his laboratory. The energy in the wire caused it to heat up quickly and shine with a brilliance that has challenged the night ever since. Once dark could be controlled, sleep was never the same.

At about the same time as the discovery of electric light, in 1880, the Industrial Revolution created factories and foundries for the production of steel and consumer goods. The furnaces in these huge factories took so long to heat up and cool off that it soon became obvious that operating them twenty-four hours a day made good business sense; shift work was born.

Today, almost 25 per cent of the work force is involved in shift work, and though twelve-hour shifts are still quite common, there are many other variations of shift work, including that of working 'on call'.

THE PROBLEM WITH SHIFT WORK

How did shift work bring Peter to his knees? Though he is an extreme example, the answer is simply that it made him chronically sleep deprived.

Before his promotion, Peter worked straight day shifts at the factory, as a machine operator. His promotion to supervisor meant that he had to begin working the night shift. Of course he was proud to be chosen as supervisor, and the salary was much better, so he accepted the job without hesitation.

It soon became evident, however, that Peter just couldn't sleep during the day – at least, not as well as he could at night. He enjoyed the feeling of relief at 8:00 a.m. as he drove away from the factory after the long shift, and he was certainly tired enough when he arrived home, but he felt he had to drive the boys to school, and then had to share a cup of coffee and breakfast with his wife before he could actually lie down to try to go to sleep.

He'd adjusted his bedroom so that it was darker, but, of course, the room wasn't pitch-black so it took him a while to fall asleep. No matter what he did, he couldn't seem to stop sunlight sneaking in.

His wife tried to keep the noise in the house to a minimum, but the telephone would ring or a neighbour would run a lawn mower, or some other unregulatable sound would startle Peter awake. He usually slept fitfully until early afternoon, then got up and attended to the chores around the house, until the boys got home from school. He took his responsibilities as a father seriously and was always available when his boys needed driving to their various sporting events or help with their homework after supper.

Later in the evening, he tried to sleep for another hour or two, and his wife would wake him at 11:00, just as she was getting ready for bed herself. As she was getting into bed, he was getting up, trying to arrive at work early just to be sure he was ahead of any potential problems.

Peter's attempts to adapt to shift work are typical, and simply reflect the difficulties shift workers have in establishing a sleep–wake cycle that matches their jobs. Remember, we all have an intrinsic biological clock that tells us when we should be asleep and when we should be awake, and this clock is set or programmed to the daylight and the dark in our everyday life. Switching from one shift to another confuses this clock.

For weeks Peter had been waking up at 7:00 a.m., having breakfast in the bright sunlight, working all morning, having lunch, working the rest of the afternoon, having supper, and going to sleep at 11:00 p.m., in complete darkness. This was his own sleep–wake cycle, and his body was used to it.

Suddenly a new programme was forced upon him. Instead of waking up at 7:00 a.m., he was asking his body to go to bed at that time. He was to have all his meals at completely different times, and in the dark. He was to stay awake at the time when he normally would have been sleeping. No wonder he had trouble adjusting.

The basic difficulty is that we humans cannot simply sleep at will, at any time. We have learned (as we saw from the cavemen experiments) that we have a clock inside of us, a programme that says, 'Now is the time you should feel sleepy; go to bed. Now you feel wide awake; get up.' The first night on the shift, at 3:00 a.m., your body and your wristwatch say, 'You should be asleep now,' but your foreman says, 'Stay awake – you've got four more hours to work!' That first night, if you were allowed to, you could sleep quite well at 3:00 a.m., but when 8:00 comes and you head home, you'll probably have difficulty sleeping. That's because your own biological sleep clock has, for some time before, dictated that 8:00 a.m. is the time for you to be up with the birds, awake and active. Your 'alarm' has gone off. It's that simple.

Your body will adapt to the new cycle, but the change takes some time. Studies have shown that the average shift worker adjusts his or her sleep–wake cycle by about an hour and a half per day, taking a full week to adjust to night work.

Imagine what would happen if, at that time, you suddenly switched shifts again. You would have to endure another week of sleep confusion, sleep deprivation and stress as your body adapted to the new cycle you imposed upon it. A week later, you probably would have adapted to the new cycle. If you worked yet another different shift at the end of this week, the process would repeat itself, leaving you in a perpetual state of sleep chaos. This is exactly what many shift workers endure on a regular basis.

OUT OF RHYTHM, OUT OF SORTS

In addition to the basic difficulty of adjusting the sleep–wake cycle, shift work has many other consequences that contribute to sleep loss.

First, most workers who begin a new shift do not compensate for the sleep they lose with that first shift. If a worker is on the day shift and is switched to night shift, for the first new shift he or she often stays awake all day (the usual routine) and then simply works all night, with the result that twenty-four hours go by with no sleep at all. The worker enters the change in shift with a sleep loss, a sleep deficit of seven hours. Thus, the worker is sleep deprived even before he or she tries to go to sleep on the new timing.

Second, we know that bright light (especially sunlight) is a very powerful time cue that resets our biological clock on a daily basis. This powerful sleep–wake stabilizer works in reverse in shift work. Essentially you must learn to sleep during the brightest time of day and learn to be awake in the dark – exactly the opposite of what you would do naturally. Not only does the powerful influence of the sun not help you adjust to your new schedule, it actually works against you.

In a similar vein, the timing of meals works against the new schedule – Peter had breakfast every day before he went to bed!

Another problem is that, even though about one in five workers operates on some sort of shift-rotation schedule, the rest of society still is much more active during the day than at night. Most of us would think twice about phoning someone at home at 3:00 a.m., except in an emergency. Society as a whole recognizes that the disturbance of sleep caused by the telephone call must be weighed against the importance of the call. However, for a night-shift worker, no such consideration exists – and their precious sleep is often interrupted by phone calls at 3:00 in the afternoon. It is of course not reasonable to ask all Peter's neighbours to postpone mowing their lawns until he gives them the signal that he is awake, but all his neighbours naturally avoid mowing the grass at daybreak.

The shift worker is very much out of synchrony with the rest of the human race. The word 'synchrony' itself comes from the Greek *syn*, meaning together, and *chronos*, meaning time.

Many shift workers face a sleeping dilemma each weekend. If they worked evenings or nights all week long, they often try, like Peter, to reverse to a diurnal cycle for their family when Saturday comes. Though he had been up all night on Friday, on Saturday morning Peter felt he just couldn't sleep: his duties as a father and husband required that he stay awake all day. He had to participate, to play cricket with his sons and go shopping with his wife, and he had to mow his own lawn, though he was exhausted. Of course, Saturday and Sunday evenings were the only nights he and his wife had as a couple, so he felt he had to stay awake at least until she went to bed. Their sexual relationship suffered; his wife felt that he didn't care anymore, but Peter was simply exhausted.

Other shift workers try, on weekends, to keep the same hours as their weekday shifts but find that no one else in the world is on their schedule. They find themselves isolated and alone. They're caught; they feel the need to be well rested to be able to work, but cannot enjoy family or social life if they take the time to sleep adequately.

The rotating of shifts minimizes some of these problems but brings a new set of difficulties. Workers on shift rotation cannot participate in the usual social events because they cannot guarantee they will be available. Most meetings, educational courses, sports events, and social gatherings are held at regular times, and most often in the evenings. Any long-term commitment to consistent attendance cannot be made by these workers.

The problems are even worse for women with children; demands of childrearing and housekeeping have no regard for the artificial shifts of industry. A nurse who works straight evenings will see her children for a few minutes when they come home from school each day, and for a few minutes at breakfast. Her nurturing, teaching, and loving can only be given at those short meetings and on weekends.

The Toll of Shift Work: Medical Problems

No wonder that shift workers are moodier, more tired and generally more irritable than their day-working colleagues. Like Peter, they are the victims of chronic sleep deprivation, which undermines their mood and their ability to concentrate and to enjoy life. They feel listless daily – out of sorts and cranky and, of course, sleepy. They tend to be more obese and less fit, and have more chronic headaches and more stomach problems, especially ulcers and constipation. They are less able to cope with life's stresses because they are unable to recharge themselves with restorative deep sleep. They often come to rely on alcohol and caffeine to try to regulate this sleep–wake chaos and minimize sleep loss. Peter began to use espresso coffee at 11:00 at night to jolt himself awake for his shift, and often would take a drink or two of whisky in the early morning if he couldn't fall off to sleep quickly. Both chemicals served the purpose, but ultimately both contributed to his sleep loss. Abuse of these chemicals and medicines for sleep is common among shift workers.

IT DOESN'T IMPROVE WITH AGE

As you age, your ability to adapt to the changes in shift work worsens. A fifty-year-old worker who has been able to tolerate shift work for years may begin to feel exhausted all the time, and dread the days around shift changes.

As we age, we usually shorten the length of our sleep–wake cycle to something less than twenty-four hours, so any change in this cycle becomes more demanding. Furthermore, the amount of deep sleep decreases with age, and thus becomes more precious. Any further loss of deep sleep because of a shift change makes the older shift worker more sleep deprived than her younger colleagues. It's simply a matter of the amount of time spent in this restorative phase.

Awakenings become much more frequent during aging, and generally sleep becomes less refreshing and more fragile. Getting to sleep and staying asleep are much more difficult. As the whole of shift-work performance depends upon adequate sleep, older workers are at a significant disadvantage.

Because of the difficulties discussed above, it's not too surprising to learn that accidents are far more common during the night shift, and especially in the hours between 3:00 and 5:00 a.m., when sleep is almost irresistible to some. In one study, researchers took EEG readings on nighttime workers in a paper mill. They found an incredible 20 per cent of workers actually 'fell asleep on the job' involuntarily. Their average 'snooze' was forty-five minutes and, though the workers reported that they had simply 'dozed off', the EEG indicated that for about a third of the time the workers had been in deep sleep. The consequences are obvious; vigilance is, to say the least, reduced, and accidents are quite common.

For example, the disastrous oil spill of the supertanker *Exxon Valdez* was attributed by the American National Transportation Safety Board to sleep loss. The third mate, who was piloting the huge vessel through the ice and islands of Prince William Sound, was severely sleep deprived. In a survey for the British Sleep Foundation 19 per cent of male drivers confessed to having fallen asleep at the wheel.

The Three Mile Island nuclear disaster in 1979 came about as the result of shift workers failing to recognize that a stuck valve was causing coolant water to be lost. This human error of omission occurred between 4:00 and 6:00 a.m. and caused the near meltdown of the reactor later that morning.

More recently, the nuclear plant catastrophe at Chernobyl has been officially acknowledged to have begun at 1:23 a.m. as the result of human error.

Clearly, the consequences of chronic sleep loss can be much more than irritability and fatigue.

TIPS FOR IMPROVING YOUR SLEEP WHILE ON SHIFT WORK

1. If you have a choice, try to avoid shift work, especially nights. For many people, especially those with fragile sleep or those over fifty, and for those who are 'larks' (have no difficulty in rising in the morning but can't stay awake at night), this type of work is simply not worth the sleep deprivation.

2. If you must do shift work, try working a regular shift – that is, not on a rotating schedule. We know that the body will adapt to the particular shift (though it takes some time), and the longer that you work the shift (within reason), the better your sleep will be. Once you have established your shift, try to keep your life in this rhythm, even on weekends. This avoids the confusion of a constantly adjusting sleep–wake cycle.

3. Shift rotation should be done in a forward manner; that is, day shift to afternoon or evening shift to night shift. It has been shown that it is much easier to adapt to this

progression of shifts than to the reverse (day shift to night shift to afternoons).

4. If possible, try to anticipate a shift change and minimize it by adjusting your bedtime several days before the shift begins. For example, if you work days and you antici- pate that next week you will have to work nights, try to go to bed a little later each day this week and wake up a little later in the morning.

5. Use bright light in the workplace and darkness in your bedroom to reset your internal timer.

6. Educate your co-workers, your personnel department, and your employer about shift work. Explore the possi- bilities of working different patterns of shift work. Many employees work two day shifts, two evening shifts, and then two nights before they have two full days off. The rapid change allows the sleep–wake cycle to remain essen- tially diurnal, and sleep loss is minimized.

7. Avoid excessive use of caffeine and alcohol and other hypnotics and stimulants. A short-acting hypnotic may occasionally be useful, but the possibility of addiction is significant.

8. Be sure that you maintain adequate nutrition, exercise and personal time while working on the night shift. This will minimize the stress of adjusting to the new time.

9. Anticipate decreased vigilance during the low point in your sleep–wake cycle (for example, between 3:00 and 5:00 a.m.), and take special precautions during this time. Jobs that involve heavy physical work make it much easier to stay awake. Jobs that involve boring repetitive tasks, such as watching a computer screen, are more likely to result in decreased vigilance and possible error.

10. Consider nighttime naps. We know that a short nap for the sleep deprived improves performance.

11. Educate your family, friends and relatives about your sleep needs. Most people will be sympathetic, including that neighbour who loves to mow the lawn.

TIPS FOR THOSE WHO LIVE WITH SHIFT WORKERS

1. Try to understand the importance of sleep to the shift worker.
2. Try to work together to maintain the quality and quantity of sleep. Ensure that the shift worker's sleep time is not interrupted by noise, household activity, and so on.
3. Schedule social and domestic events to coincide with the new sleep–wake cycle of the shift worker.
4. Ensure that the shift worker receives adequate nutrition and exercise. Shift workers' nutrition often suffers because their mealtimes are different from those of the rest of the family. Shift workers are prone to obesity and stomach disorders. Try to ensure that meals are regular and nourishing, despite the change in work pattern.
5. Shift work does allow for workers to be available to their families at odd hours. Use this to your advantage. For example, a night-shift worker might very well be available to attend a child's end-of-term party the next afternoon at school or an early-morning fishing trip on a weekend. Be imaginative with this special time.

On Call: A Different Kind of Shift Work

It's 4:30 a.m. and the ambulance pulls into the Casualty Department, with its lights flashing in the dark. The pyjama-clad patient is wheeled quickly inside, one arm dangling awkwardly from the stretcher, the hand open and useless to protest as an ambulance attendant pushes heavily and grotesquely against the victim's chest. There is an air of desperation and great urgency, of precious time passing quickly.

The doctor rushes into the room, dressed in a set of operating-room greens and rubbing his eyes; he's been sleeping in a room in the hospital, 'on call' for just such an emergency. Quickly the medical team works to try to save the patient's life. There is an established protocol, but decisions have to be made very rapidly, and complicated physical activities must be accomplished smoothly within seconds. There are drug dosages to be recalled, and the responsibilities are heavy. The entire team works under the direction of this physician, who only a few seconds ago was fast asleep. All the while, the consequences of failure are absolute.

One variant of shift work is that of being 'on call'. It's a common working condition among emergency personnel such as firefighters, medical workers, and the people who repair utilities. The term refers to workers who are allowed to sleep but have to be prepared to be awakened suddenly, and to function quickly thereafter, often in life-and-death situations. The employee is literally allowed to 'sleep on the job', though this type of shift work is much more demanding than it at first appears.

Sleeping While 'On Call'

From studies of physicians as well as other emergency workers 'on call', we know that sleep is poor during these shifts – in some cases as bad as no sleep at all.

First, the total amount of sleep is reduced. Obviously, if you are awakened at all, the amount of time spent asleep is less, but also the length of time that it takes to fall asleep is very much increased for many 'on call' workers. It's as if the tranquility, the peace, that allows them to fall off to sleep is threatened by the idea that they may be awakened at any time. Such workers often insist on going to bed later than usual, preferring this to the annoying feeling of being called as soon as they drift off.

Returning to sleep after being awakened for an emergency is very difficult indeed – simply because the emotional response to the event is so marked.

'On call' sleep is different in quality from normal sleep. In general, it involves much less deep sleep, and decreased REM sleep. Repeated awakenings, if frequent enough, prevent the sleeper from entering deep sleep at all. Each time they're awakened and try to return to sleep, 'on call' workers must progress through the twilight zones to achieve deep sleep, but just as they get to this restorative phase, the telephone rings again. Interestingly, even if you are not called at all over the shift, your sleep is different. In general, it is much lighter than normal sleep, and includes much more twilight-zone sleep. It's as if the anticipation of being called is enough in itself to block adequate relaxation; you simply can't have a normal restful sleep.

If you have managed to achieve deep sleep and are called, you must rise up from the full depth of this sleep to consciousness. Your mind doesn't work well for a few minutes; you're foggy and slower than usual, even a bit confused. This has obvious consequences in some jobs, such as that of the physician in the Accident and Emergency department.

BEING 'ON CALL' IS MUCH MORE COMMON THAN YOU THINK

Many groups in society who would not normally wear paging devices or consider themselves 'on call' are, in fact, exactly that during sleep – available for crises or problems that might arise during the night.

You have an eight-year-old daughter who seemed well during the day but who began to run a fever after supper.

You gave her some medicine for fever and put her to bed, and you've just gone in to check on her before you yourself head off to sleep. She is flushed and coughing, she looks ill, she feels hot again.

How well will you sleep tonight? You will in fact be 'on call' – resting lightly, your senses tuned to your daughter's needs. Chances are you will never enter deep sleep at all, but will spend much of the evening in twilight-zone sleep. In the morning, you will be sleep deprived.

This situation is quite common among other groups as well. Family members of disabled persons, mothers and fathers waiting for their teenagers to return from late outings, anyone with elderly parents living at home – in short, many in society who have responsibility for the care of others – are all 'on call'. Even if they are never called, the anticipation is enough to make them chronically sleep deprived. Essentially, their perception of the environment is heightened, enabling them to respond to the need. This increased awareness interferes with their sleep, even if they are not actually awakened. Obviously, if they are called and their sleep is disrupted, the sleep deprivation becomes even more marked.

Tips for Sleeping 'On Call'

1. Realize the toll that being 'on call' takes. Take the time to replace the sleep lost; do not simply carry on. Even if you are never called, your sleep will be less refreshing. If you don't replace the sleep that is lost, your performance and your mood will suffer.

2. Try to avoid repeated awakenings. Instruct anyone who must call you to accumulate the calls, saving them up so that you may deal with several problems at once. Obviously this depends upon the nature of the problem,

but try to avoid being awakened for minor difficulties again and again.

3. Don't try to force a return to sleep. If the response to the call has been significant, it may naturally take you some time to be able to fall asleep again. Use this time profitably to relax or accomplish something else rather than fighting to try to sleep.

4. Avoid stimulants and caffeine to try to jolt you awake when called. They only make it more difficult to get to sleep again.

5. Don't mix up your time cues. If you are called out at night, don't spend a long time outside enjoying the sunrise when you should be catching up on your lost sleep. Try not to eat much when you're awakened; stick to fruit juices and light snacks if you're hungry, for the same reason.

6. Realize the limitations of functioning after quickly awakening from deep sleep. If possible, give yourself some time to be able to function normally.

7. Being 'on call' informally, as are the parents of a newborn child, is a demanding experience. Recognize that you may very well have a limit as to how much of this you can take without your mood and your performance suffering. A regular break from this responsibility helps. Accept that in this circumstance, because the quality of your sleep is different, you might very well need to sleep longer. Consider napping during the day to minimize sleep deprivation.

Jet Lag

Suppose that, one night, just as you were slipping on your pyjamas to go to sleep, you were by some magical process lifted up out of your bedroom and transported far away, to another land. And just suppose that, when you arrived in the far-off place, everyone was just waking up! Wouldn't it be fun? Wouldn't it be wonderful? Wouldn't it be very, very tiring?

This is exactly what happens to millions of people around the world every year with modern jet travel. After boarding a darkened aeroplane in the early evening at home, passengers fly for only a few hours and then arrive, often having had no sleep at all, at the beginning of a new day in a brand-new world. Not surprisingly, they feel fatigued even as they walk down the exit ramp from the aeroplane. Modern air travel is a wearying method of transportation, and there are many reasons for flight passengers' fatigue. Not the least is the micro-environment in which they have flown.

The noise and vibration of the plane, as well as the cramped seating, usually prevent effective sleep. Passengers complain of sore muscles as the confined seating space and aisles prevent movement and stretching of the limbs. Because of reduced barometric pressure (the cabins are depressurized to 8,000 feet or 2400 metres), the concentration of oxygen available to passengers for the duration of the flight is much lower than they were used to at sea level. The air circulating in the cabin holds as much oxygen as is present at the very top of a 8,000-foot (2.4-kilometre) mountain. This air also has a very low humidity (sometimes as low as 5 per cent), causing red and irritated eyes and dry mucous membranes in the nose and throat. The anxiety that flying frequently causes may very well have prompted the passenger to have an alcoholic drink or two or even a sedative. All these factors can contribute to a traveller's weariness upon entering the bustle of the airport at his or her destination.

Daylight Saving Time: Jet Lag for the Masses

Every year, over 850 million people around the world, in twenty-five countries, have jet lag thrust upon them when they switch their clocks to daylight saving time or 'summer time'. Originally conceived by Benjamin Franklin as a method of giving more hours of daylight to the working day, it was introduced in the UK in 1916. The technique of advancing the clock by one hour in the spring, then setting it back by one hour in the autumn, is equivalent to crossing a time zone in an aeroplane.

Studies have shown that the adjustment takes most people about a week, and has significant effects on mood, performance and accident rates. The springtime, or forward, shift is more difficult than the delaying autumnal shift because the inherent sleep–wake cycle adjusts better to a lengthening of the day, since the cycle itself is slightly longer than twenty-four hours. As might be expected, there is increased irritability on awakening during the adjustment week, particularly in spring. Most people feel less alert, less calm and less well rested. The incidence of motor-vehicle accidents is increased by almost 8 per cent in the week after the spring shift. In contrast, after the autumn shift, most people feel they have benefited from the extra hour of sleep; they are calmer, and there is no significant change in the accident rate.

TRAVELLER'S TIME WARP

But it is, after all, a brand-new place and a brand-new day. When you arrive after an overnight flight across several time zones, your surroundings and the people you meet all say, 'Good morning', but your wristwatch and your body say, 'Good night'. Succumbing to your own internal clock, you try to grab a couple of listless hours of sleep in a hotel room, but you are eager not to miss any of your holiday, so are soon out enjoying the afternoon. You are so tired that you can hardly wait to go to bed, and so arrange to hit the sack early, only to wake up in the wee hours of the morning local time, unable to go back to sleep. You spend the next four or five days adjusting to the new schedule, all the while feeling fatigued and sleepy and unable to concentrate. You complain of headaches, constipation and nausea. Above all, you're irritable – you're not as happy as you thought you would be, and your performance is less than optimal. Welcome to jet lag – a supreme example of how important the rhythms, the cycles within us, are to our well-being.

Face it: your own internal rhythms cannot adjust quickly. It's not the jet that lags behind – it's you! Specifically, your sleep–wake cycle takes a while to adjust to a new dawn and dusk. Remember, we human beings simply cannot sleep whenever we wish. In evolutionary terms, we never had to before, until rapid air transportation made it possible to cross time zones quickly. The modern air passenger's internal timing system continues on the old pattern until it is reset, or readjusted, by new time cues in the new environment.

There are two major modifying factors for the symptoms of jet lag, factors that can make the symptoms better or worse: the number of time zones crossed and the direction of flight.

The world is divided into twenty-four time zones, approximately 15 degrees of longitude apart. Each of these zones is an hour different from those on each side of it. Obviously, crossing one time zone does not produce as much of a phase shift in your sleep–wake cycle as crossing five will. Travelling all the way around the earth on one flight would cause no time-zone shift. Travelling north/south does not produce jet lag because no time zones are crossed.

A passenger's system readjusts more quickly after westward flight than eastward flight. This phenomenon has been measured: travellers on average adjust one hour a day for eastward flights, and one-and-a-half hours a day for westward flights. Why is this so? The answer lies in the sleep–wake cycle. The discrepancy reflects the fact that the human biological clock has an inherent tendency to lengthen its period beyond twenty-four hours – to lengthen its 'day'. Westward flight does exactly this: it lengthens the day. Flights to the east shorten the day. For example, if you took off from London at 9:00 p.m. and arrived in Sri Lanka at 8:00 a.m. your 'night' would be six hours shorter than it would have been if you had stayed in the airport. Because the circadian sleep–wake cycle tends to be longer than twenty-four hours, the westward-flight adaptation is easier; it conforms to your own tendency. Remember the scientists in the cave who automatically went to bed an hour later each day? If your flight is westward, and only crosses one time zone, you would go to bed one hour later that day too. This conforms with your basic tendency to lengthen the day. If you travel eastward, however, it would be like asking the scientists in the cave to go to bed an hour earlier – the opposite of their natural tendency.

Suppose you are travelling by aeroplane, not simply for a holiday but because you have an important business meeting, a meeting that demands all your skill as a communicator and salesperson and all your social abilities. Or suppose you have to travel across several time zones because you are an athlete competing in an international event like the Olympics. Imagine that you are a commander of the armed forces having to transport fairly large numbers of military personnel across several time zones for a strategic manoeuvre during wartime.

In all these examples, the ability to minimize the effects of jet lag might very well mean the difference between success or failure, winning or losing, life or death.

Because three out of four travellers who cross three time zones or more have significant symptoms of jet lag, an understanding of its causes and of ways to remedy it is very important.

Tips for Minimizing Jet Lag

1. Try to anticipate the change. Over several nights before your trip, move your sleeping and eating schedule towards the time in your destination. Do this gradually; you don't have to do it completely, but any move that you make approximating the new time schedule will minimize the effects of jet lag. For example, if you will be travelling from Europe to Asia, advance the time at which you retire at night and awaken the next morning prior to departure. Begin by advancing the time you go to bed by twenty minutes or half an hour, and do this each night for several nights.

2. Try not to arrive at your destination sleep-deprived. If possible, sleep well the night before you travel. If the flight takes place during your usual sleep time, do your best to sleep on the aeroplane.

3. Try to drink lots of fluid during the flight. Dehydration makes it more difficult to adjust to a new time schedule. Avoid alcohol because it alters the sleep pattern. Avoid caffeine and other stimulant-containing beverages because these only serve to confuse your sleep–wake cycle further.

4. If you came to attend an important meeting or a performance, or you must be at your best for whatever reason, there is no substitute for arriving several days early to acclimatize, or at least to minimize the effects of jet lag. Arrange the meeting for a time that suits your sleep–wake cycle. If you fly overnight from Europe to Asia and attend a meeting at 10:00 the next morning, your body and your mind will be asleep.

5. Whenever you arrive, switch to the new time right away. Go outside and get some sunshine, as bright daylight is one of the best time cues. Adopt new mealtimes and

sleeping hours quickly. Jet-lag symptoms last longer in people who stay inside, in their dark hotel rooms, than in people who are outside in natural light.

6. Though there is still some debate, most studies agree that changes in diet do not help to minimize jet-lag symptoms.

7. If you must sleep on arrival, sleep only a short time, two hours or less.

8. If you are travelling through time zones very quickly or through several time zones in a very short time, sometimes it's better not to shift zones at all, but simply to keep your cycle on home time.

9. If all else fails, using a short-acting hypnotic (see Chapter 11) for a short period may help reset your sleep–wake cycle.

10. A promising possibility is a hormone called melatonin. It's produced by the pineal gland in the base of your brain exclusively at night. In experiments, the hormone was given in tablet form and literally tricked the body into altering its internal clock. Although this is not licensed in the UK, it may be prescribed by a specialist.

Seasonal Affective Disorder

Do you find yourself depressed every winter? When the days shorten and the nights get dark and long, do you find yourself losing energy – sleeping longer hours but feeling less refreshed? Do you eat more during the dark winter months? If so, you may have seasonal affective disorder (SAD), a result of your affect (or feelings) and your sleep pattern changing with the lack of sunlight.

If you lived at the equator, each day would be exactly

Melatonin: The Hormone of Darkness

As animals, we humans have evolved mechanisms to ensure our ability to survive even under the most dramatic of environmental extremes.

We know that many of our physiological functions vary from season to season – how do the cells within our bodies recognize that the daylight hours are changing?

The answer seems to be that this information is sent to each of the cells in our bodies via the hormone melatonin (the word comes from the Greek *melas*, meaning black or dark).

The hormone melatonin is secreted by the pineal gland, a small down-pouching of the brain that is situated directly behind the eyes. The anatomical connection to the eyes is not accidental – the main control for the secretion of melatonin comes from the eyes, and specifically from the effect of bright light such as sunshine on the retina. Melatonin is barely secreted at all during the daylight hours, but the levels in the bloodstream rise quickly as the sun sets, and they reach their peak at about midnight or soon thereafter. This secretion occurs whether or not the person sleeps, and the secretion can be altered by light – exposure to bright light of whatever source (sunlight or artificial light) causes the melatonin secretion to dwindle quickly to daytime levels. Melatonin, then, is the 'hormone of darkness' in humans, just as it is in other animals, even nocturnal ones such as bats.

Melatonin is quickly distributed through the bloodstream to every single cell in the body, and thus every part of us knows whether or not it is dark outside even if that particular cell, or organ, or tissue, cannot 'see' whether or not the sun is shining, or the days are getting shorter. Melatonin is, then, a chemical messenger, telling all the different parts of our body that it's nighttime, or, indirectly, that winter is coming.

Melatonin itself has a sedative effect, and causes us to be sleepy – but this effect is only mild. It also has an effect to lower body temperature slightly, which is helpful in initiating sleep. Thus the hormone has the effect of telling the entire body whether or not it's light outside, and, if light is absent, the hormone has the effect of decreasing arousal and increasing the propensity to sleep by beginning to lower temperature. But melatonin has many other effects. It is known to be a biological moderator of mood, sexual behaviour, circadian rhythms and the functioning of the immune system.

twelve hours long and each night the same all year long. Most of us do not live on this narrow strip girdling the earth, so we experience times of the year when the days are longer.

Sunlight is the most powerful *Zeitgeber*, or time cue, and for some people lack of sunlight produces a feeling of fatigue, depression and altered sleep pattern every winter. They are literally SAD – withdrawn, moody, irritable and lethargic, and lacking ambition and motivation. They sleep long hours. Their appetite increases, especially for sweets and starchy foods, and they put on weight.

The condition was first described in a woman who had severe depression every single year, but only in the wintertime. She lived, over the years, in several different cities in the northern part of the United States, and no matter where she lived, her melancholy would return every winter and her symptoms would disappear each spring. One year, she took a Caribbean holiday and, within two days of being in the bright equatorial sunshine, her depression began to improve. Her psychiatrist, reasoning that the sunlight was an important difference in the locations, suggested that the lack of sunlight might be the operative cause. He tested this hypothesis by treating her with daily exposure to a bank of bright fluorescent lights once she returned to her northern city. He was able to treat her depression and prevent its recurrence by the regular use of this fluorescent light every winter.

The understanding now is that this phenomenon is common, and severe depression is probably just the tip of the iceberg. Many people experience a change in their mood, sleep patterns and weight over the months when the sunlight hours are decreased. Only a relatively small number of this large group have severe symptoms, but many are affected to a lesser degree. Their symptoms appear in the autumn and clear up spontaneously by springtime in northern climates. It seems that the feeble light of the winter sun is simply not adequate for these people to reset their own sleep–wake cycle daily. They are allowed essentially free rein – like the scientists in the cave – and the resulting sleep problem is associated with the mood change.

To control the problem, bright light is all that is needed. Sunlight is best, but of course it's not available when the symptoms appear. Regular indoor light is not intense enough, so special light boxes that simulate sunlight have been used with good results. SAD may be caused by excess production of melatonin, a hormone secreted by the pineal gland during periods of darkness. It is the same hormone that is responsible for the hibernation behaviour of some mammals. The secretion of melatonin is inhibited by light, and large doses of melatonin injected intravenously can produce sleepiness and lethargy as well as depression.

Light must be fairly bright – mimicking bright sunlight – to treat seasonal affective disorder. The scientific measurement of intensity of light is called 'lux', and midday sunlight is about 100,000 lux. A normal room's lighting level is about 250–500 lux. Light therapy for SAD usually uses a light source that produces at least 2,500 lux.

It is suspected that millions of people around the world experience some change in their mood and performance as the days shorten. In extremes such as the Arctic, where continuous darkness persists for several months each year, the lack of sunlight and the consequent changes in mood and sleeping patterns are well-known stress factors. Appreciation of this biological phenomenon may well make you feel happier during the long winter months.

Tips for Dealing with Seasonal Affective Disorder

1. Use natural light to your advantage – even if the daylight hours are shortened, sunshine is the best rhythm setter. Go for a walk; time outside activity to the period of

The Big Chill: The Sleep of Hibernation

Many of us do not like the long cold nights of winter, and the freezing temperatures and reduced daytime sunlight often make us lethargic. Our evenings are dark and less active than in the summer, and our nightly sleeping time is increased. In some other animals, the response to these environmental changes is even more marked and the phenomenon of hibernation, a period of reduced physical activity and lowered body temperature, is often seen. Hibernation has evolved as an adaptive behaviour to allow these animals to survive extremely inhospitable climates. Hibernation is particularly common in cold-blooded animals, those that have no source of internal heat, such as reptiles. These creatures depend on external sources for their heat – usually the sun, the warm earth and air – and as the ambient temperature begins to fall in autumn, and the hours of daylight become less (both stimuli seem to be important), these animals begin to store food in anticipation of their long winter's sleep. As the days shorten more, they find a protected environment, lower their body temperature, and enter a state of suspended animation – including a drowsy state of reduced consciousness that very much resembles deep sleep. This allows them to survive over the extremely cold winter period as their metabolic needs are much reduced.

They do not actually freeze – the formation of ice crystals in their tissues would kill them, but many of them maintain their temperatures only half a degree centigrade or so above freezing. Frogs, salamanders and turtles are often completely surrounded by ice when they hibernate, and the Alaska black fish is actually solidly encased in ice throughout the long Arctic winter. Many insects spend the winter in a similar state of hibernation, often in a larval or pupal stage, and butterflies and moths hibernate in their cocoons. Even the pesky mosquito, after its last feeding in autumn, hibernates over the winter subsisting on stored food.

Though hibernation is quite common in cold-blooded animals, many warm-blooded animals hibernate as well. Bats survive over the period of winter, when food supplies are scarce and food gathering difficult, by huddling together on the roofs of caves or other protected environments. Their core temperature drops, and they remain immobile, sometimes for weeks. Hibernation allows animals to conserve energy – it decreases the metabolic rate to less than one-thirtieth of that of the same animal at rest in ambient temperatures – a tremendous energy saving!

There is a theory that deep sleep in humans has evolved to allow us a prolonged period of energy conservation each night. We may have evolved our own pattern of daily hibernation.

maximum light; open a curtain or blind – enjoy what precious sunlight is available.

2. Use bright light to encourage a regular sleep–wake cycle both at home and at work. Skylights, large windows, and bright artificial light may very well improve your mood and performance.

3. Buy or build a light source. Commercial lamps are available at reasonable prices, or you can build your own. Use two 4-foot (120-centimetre) fluorescent tubes with some sort of diffuser in front to absorb the glare. Place the light source in a spot where it will be easy for you to be exposed to it.

4. As the dark is a stressor to your sleep–wake cycle, try to keep other stressors to a minimum. Keep a regular schedule of retiring, and especially awakening; keep up your physical activity; watch your intake of caffeine and alcohol. The single most important factor in resetting your sleep–wake cycle over the winter is probably a regular wake-up time.

5. If you can find the ways and means to travel to a source of bright sunlight, enjoy it. A week or two away during the darkest period of winter can improve your sense of well-being tremendously.

3

Sleep Deprivation, Snoring and Sleep Apnoea

You're tired. Your eyes burn as if they have been rubbed with steel wool. Dim light or shade helps somewhat, but the bright sunshine of morning makes you squint and wince in pain. The dryness, the grittiness, are unrelenting; your poor eyes are so tired that they cannot even produce enough tears for their own comfort. It's very difficult to keep your eyes open, and when they do close, even for a brief wink of time, the soothing relief is immediate.

The rest of your body is unhappy as well. Your head throbs its displeasure – not an acute stabbing pain but a steady, wearying, punishing ache. You feel cold, perhaps nauseated, and certainly weak. It's an effort to move, and only a conscious act of will overcomes the inertia.

Mentally you're no longer the happy-go-lucky person you are when well rested. Your zest for life has vanished, leaving a much paler spirit behind, who asks only to be left alone, to sleep. You're irritable, moody, and you're closer to tears than usual. Everything seems to require much more effort.

Face it, you're miserable.

No wonder sleep deprivation, the extreme on the insomnia continuum, was used as a torture during the Spanish Inquisition.

We all spend about one-third of our life asleep; if you live to be eighty, that works out to about twenty-seven years of sleeping.

Sleep is, quite simply, a biological necessity, a demanding human need that must be met by most of us daily, just like the need for food to eat, water to drink, and air to breathe.

Faced with this imposed biological sentence of sleep, many have tried to shorten the time needed for rest, and their observations are important in helping us to understand this basic daily requirement.

Randy Gardner: A Boy with a Dream

In January 1965, Randy Gardner was a seventeen-year-old San Diego high school student with a problem: he didn't have a project for his high school science fair. He wasn't interested in the usual sorts of science projects, but wanted to do something 'extreme'.

Randy chose for himself a most unusual science project: he decided to try to qualify for entry into the famous *Guinness Book of World Records*. The achievement he was after was in the field of endurance. The challenge was straightforward – all he had to do was stay awake.

He wanted to be able to lay claim to the longest documented time without any sleep at all, to stay awake longer than anyone else had ever done in the past. The old record in the book was 260 hours of continuous wakefulness. He was going to try to beat it. To make his mark, Randy would

Can We Learn to Sleep Less?

'Sleep,' said Thomas Edison, 'is a colossal waste of time.'

Experiments have been done with volunteers who tried to reduce their sleep from the usual seven and a half hours to five and a half hours by decreasing their sleep by thirty minutes every two weeks. Most of the volunteers had little trouble reducing sleep by a half-hour, or even an hour, but they began to notice some difficulty when sleep was reduced by more than this. They were able to awaken on time, and they were able to function at work and in their social obligations, but they found themselves simply more fatigued. The sleep reduction didn't seem to pose a threat to anyone's health, and the extra time was useful for studying, exercising or watching television. However, many of them just 'didn't feel as well'. They found themselves to be more irritable, more pessimistic and less fun to be with, though often their co-workers and peers did not notice much of a change.

All the volunteers had difficulty in reducing their sleep beyond five and a half hours a night. This may be a biological limit for most adults. Most of the volunteers increased the amount of sleep they obtained when the study was over.

For most adults, reduction in the amount of sleep is possible, but fatigue and changes in mood make it undesirable. It is estimated that about half of the adult North American population is already sleep deprived (that is, receiving less than the ideal amount of sleep), and any further reduction would have marked changes on mood, vigilance and performance. In the UK about 11 per cent of adult drivers have fallen asleep at least once when driving, most commonly due to simple sleep restriction.

simply have to stay awake for eleven days, with no rest at all, no naps, no breaks.

Randy found that the first couple of days (and nights) weren't too difficult at all. He enlisted the help of a couple of friends, who kept him awake at night by walking, playing games or doing other exercise, talking, or even by goading him to take cold showers. Randy vowed to use no kind of stimulant throughout the science project, not even coffee. The first night was easy. By the end of the second day, though, he did feel quite tired; he had trouble focusing his eyes and couldn't read. Soon afterwards he was unable to watch television – the images were too blurred – and that symptom remained for the rest of the experiment. His eyelids became so heavy that he spent the rest of the time tilting his head back to see.

By the third day, his mood was definitely different – he was irritable and wanted to be left alone. He had trouble with coordination, and there was some slurring of his speech.

On the fourth day, he became more than irritable – he became uncooperative. He began to have lapses of memory, which would occur more and more frequently as time went on. He complained of seeing 'fog' around streetlamps, and believed that someone's tweed suit was made of worms. The prolonged sleeplessness was obviously taking its toll, but he would not give in and close his eyes to sleep.

By the end of five days, Randy's parents were worried that the prolonged lack of sleep might cause him some psychological harm – that he might become mentally ill, truly insane – from lack of sleep. They had some cause for concern.

Six years earlier, in New York City, a disc jockey named Peter Tripp had, in fact, become mentally ill after attempting a similar stretch of sleeplessness. Tripp's continuous sleeplessness was a publicity stunt, to raise money for the March of Dimes, a large American charity. He broadcast a daily programme from Times Square, and crowds gathered to watch him in his glass booth. By using stimulants, he was able to stay awake for two hundred continuous hours (about nine days), but in the last few nights of his sleeplessness he became paranoid and his behaviour resulted in the marathon being stopped. It appeared that lack of sleep had made him insane, at least temporarily.

Randy's experience was generally much better than the radio announcer's. Despite a few hallucinations, he never manifested serious symptoms of psychiatric disorder, and was always in touch with reality.

By the end of nine full days of sleeplessness, however, major effects of sleep loss began to be noticeable in Randy. He could no longer speak in full sentences, but used only fragmented collections of phrases. He had frequent memory lapses and difficulty following conversations. It appeared that he was paying attention only part of the time and had an obvious inability to concentrate. Nevertheless, he was still determined to succeed.

On the last evening, even though his vision was very poor and he often saw double, he chose to try to stay awake by spending part of the time at an all-night penny arcade, playing a basketball game. Randy played against his attendant for the evening, the renowned sleep researcher Dr William Dement, and though he had been awake continuously for almost 250 hours and Dr Dement had had regular sleep, Randy won every one of the hundred games they played!

The next day, Randy did indeed break the old record, with a new figure of 264 hours of continuous wakefulness, eleven full days and nights without sleep.

When he went to bed later that day, after his stint of 264 hours of wakefulness, researchers had no idea how long he might sleep to make up for the hours of rest that he had missed. Surprisingly, he slept only fourteen hours and forty minutes that night, and the following night only eight hours. Within several nights, he was back to his usual pattern of sleeping – about seven to seven and a half hours a night. He never made up the eleven nights' sleep he had lost.

Throughout the whole ordeal, Randy demonstrated no marked abnormal psychological or physical symptoms, except for a few mild hallucinations. He suffered no lasting emotional or physical damage, and after several nights' normal rest, appeared to have recovered completely.

The Mental and Physical Effects of Sleep Deprivation

Most of us don't try to stay awake for eleven days straight as Randy did. What happens is not that we avoid sleeping altogether, but rather that we accumulate a sleep debt and try to function on less than the optimal amount.

Say you need seven and a half hours of sleep a night to feel alert on awakening and not excessively sleepy during the day, but that work pressures or other factors such as illness or anxiety prevent you from getting more than six hours a night. By the end of a week you have accumulated seven hours of sleep debt – a full night's worth. You are probably not hallucinating, not seeing fog around lampposts or imagining that tweed jackets are woven out of worms – in fact, you are unlikely to experience any of the dramatic effects of complete sleep loss. However, you are not quite the same as you would have been had you slept as long as you needed. This is the common type of sleep deprivation, and the one we have all experienced.

Mood is one of the first casualties of sleep loss. In general, when you have been deprived of sleep, your emotional reserve is markedly diminished, making you less adaptable. Events seem to take more of a toll on your feelings than they would if you were well rested. You are much more likely to feel saddened, depressed and forlorn. Fatigue and hopelessness are all-pervasive.

Feelings of persecution, of mild paranoia, often develop after seventy-two hours or more of sleep loss. However, only in 2 to 3 per cent of cases do gross psychiatric changes (such as those experienced by Peter Tripp) appear, even after prolonged sleep loss.

Motivation often diminishes quickly with sleep loss. Though there is very little measurable difference in dexterity or manual performance, the willingness to attend to even simple tasks wanes. If you are tested on mathematical skills or chess moves, sleep loss doesn't seem to make much difference. What is different, though, is that you're simply not interested in doing the math or playing chess; you'd rather rest. Studies of sleep loss among soldiers in the Israeli Army produced interesting results. A cardinal rule for these soldiers is to fill up their canteens with water at every opportunity. It's a basic rule for surviving the climate in the Middle East. After manoeuvres involving some sleep loss, Israeli soldiers were able to shoot just as accurately and perform other military tasks just as well, but the essential principle of replacing water reserves was simply forgotten, as though the motivation for survival had vanished. The same phenomenon is observable among overtired junior hospital doctors; they are able to keep up with often complicated drug regimens but sometimes will skip that extra walk down the corridor and around the wards to check on their patients.

Tasks that involve forethought, planning and anticipation are the ones that suffer when you are deprived of sleep. It's as if your perspective changes, and you lose grasp of the relative importance of actions. Your ability to reason and think remains relatively unaffected, but your desire, your will, is diminished.

Higher neurological functions are impaired by sleep loss as well. The first observable change is usually a decrease in your awareness of your environment, and your perception of differences slows. This change has grave consequences for those employed as professional lorry drivers or power-plant supervisors who monitor computer screens, for in these situations extreme vigilance must be exercised while doing fairly boring, repetitive tasks.

When you are deprived of sleep, your eyes don't work as well, and difficulties with vision are very common. The first changes are usually minor: some blurring of vision when reading, or some errors in judging distance or depth. You may reach for a tea cup and miss because your eyes told you it was closer. As the period without sleep lengthens, other visual errors become more common. Though a significant number of normal people who undergo extended periods of wakefulness have hallucinations, it usually takes a prolonged sleep loss – at least seventy-two hours – to bring these on. During sleep loss of shorter duration, visual errors, mistakes in vision, are much more common. Perhaps you 'saw' the doorknob on the left rather than the right, or misread the hands on the clock. These errors don't happen if you focus your mind specifically on the doorknob, for example, but if you are looking at something else and glimpse the door out of the corner of your eye, your perception of the knob's location may very well be wrong if you are very sleepy. These errors are easily corrected, and often comical, but they do show that the visual system, one of the most important for information gathering, is not working well. Similarly, it's quite common to have some difficulty with coordination, and mild hand tremor or difficulty with fine motor skills (such as threading a needle) often occurs.

One of the most consistent findings in studies of prolonged sleep loss is impairment of memory, especially memory of recent events. Somehow the system of committing information to memory, which is a very complicated process, does not work at all well when we have lost sleep. For this reason, it is more difficult to learn new information when you are sleep deprived. The system whereby your brain assimilates knowledge and then keeps it available for retrieval (that's really all memory is) just doesn't function nearly as well when you are not well rested.

Everything Hurts When You Don't Sleep

Physically – apart from being sleepy, of course – several changes occur when you are deprived of sleep. There is no doubt that you are more sensitive to pain. Many so-called chronic pain syndromes, such as fibromyalgia, are associated with daily sleep loss, and this poor quality of sleep is felt to be part of the cause of the pain; sensitivity to pain is known to be heightened even after short periods of sleep loss. Consider the following experiment. Volunteers were exposed to several painful stimuli and asked to grade them in severity. For example, a blood pressure cuff was inflated on the arm and the volunteer had to say whether it was mildly uncomfortable, extremely uncomfortable or unbearable at a particular pressure. After several nights of relatively minor sleep deprivation, almost all the volunteers felt pain at a lower pressure of the cuff compressing their arm. Pain is, of course, a purely subjective feeling, but there is evidence to suggest that you feel pain much more easily when you're tired. This is important news for anyone who has chronic pain.

Increased appetite is a common symptom of sleep deprivation, though the mechanism is not understood. Could it be that chronic sleep loss contributes to the epidemic of obesity? It certainly is possible that one is related to the other.

In a similar vein, increased sexual drive is often a symptom of sleep loss. This is surprising, because most physical stresses

Sleep After Sex

Most people, both male and female, are aware of an increased tendency towards sleep after sexual orgasm. The feeling of muscular relaxation, the intimacy, and the calm or peace that is often present after orgasm – all contribute to encourage the onset of sleep.

This tendency to sleep after sex is often more pronounced in men. Norepinephrine, a neurotransmitter involved in the body's sympathetic nervous system, is present in men in large amounts during intercourse, but the level falls soon afterwards. Because this chemical has an alerting effect, men feel sleepier as the level drops.

However, sexual activity that does not lead to orgasm may very well make sleep nearly impossible. The heightened sensory awareness, feelings of frustration or anger, and interpersonal conflicts that often result when only one partner reaches orgasm contribute to a delay in the arrival of sleep, and in fact make sleep, when it does come, lighter and interrupted by frequent awakenings. It seems clear, then, that sexual intercourse itself is not the cause for increased sleepiness, but orgasm. Some sexual activity that does not lead directly to orgasm may be very relaxing – for example, massage, stroking, light touch or simple physical closeness such as hugging. These activities, which reinforce interpersonal bonds and communicate emotions between people, allow us to relax, and to let sleep occur.

cause a decrease in sexual drive, a reduction that makes sense from an evolutionary point of view; the process of mating is threatened by any physical force that would decrease one's ability to care for offspring. Nevertheless, chronic sleep loss can produce increased libido.

MICROSLEEPS: HERE ONE MINUTE, GONE THE NEXT

How does your mind cope with enforced sleep loss? If you insist that it must stay awake, what does it do?

With significant sleep deprivation, your brain recognizes that it needs some rest, and in spite of whatever else you're trying to do, sleep will occur, but only for a few seconds at a time. These short bursts of sleep, documented on EEGs, are called 'microsleeps'; they're universal among those who have experienced prolonged sleep deprivation. These microsleeps are forced on you; you don't ask for them, but they intrude onto your wakefulness anyway, barging in and taking control of your mind for a second or two at a time. They consist mainly of Stage I (light or twilight-zone) sleep, and thus they allow your brain some rest even when you are not in bed. Of course, even though you're not wide awake for the several seconds of microsleep, you don't lose muscle control and fall down; nevertheless, your mind is not aware of the external environment for those few seconds – remember, that's the definition of sleep. After a short pause in brain functioning, your brain works normally again, and you are wide awake and fully responsive. This lapse means that, if someone had been speaking to you, you would have missed a word or two. If you were involved in a boring, repetitive task (say, adding up figures on an adding machine), you might 'forget' to add one or two figures, or momentarily lose your place in the column. What's more, you would not be aware that this was going on. If the task at hand needed all your concentration, microsleeps would not occur, but when performing low-stimulus, tedious, repetitive tasks, the brain readily allows microsleeps, and without your being aware of it you are here one minute and gone the next. The significance of this to jobs that require alertness is obvious – it can be disastrous!

THE RAT RACE

Is it possible to go without sleep completely? Probably not. We do know that experimental animals who are not allowed to sleep at all will eventually die, though we are not exactly sure why. This evidence comes from an experiment with laboratory rats done by sleep researcher Alan Rechtschaffen in Chicago in 1983. He showed that sleep deprivation was uniformly fatal for these animals. In the experiment, he had electrodes implanted in the brains of two rats so he could identify, by EEG, when the rats were sleeping. Then the animals were placed in a Plexiglas cylinder with a clear partition separating them; they were visible to each other and to the experimenter. The bottom of the cage consisted of a circular floor attached to a motor that rotated it. Both rats had access to water and food.

While the control rat was allowed to sleep as much as he liked, whenever the experimental rat tried to sleep, the motor would come on, and the base of the cage would turn. Because the rat had to walk (to keep from banging into the side of the cage) as the floor beneath it rotated, the animal was effectively prohibited from obtaining any sleep whatsoever. He was stuck in a real rat race.

No startling differences were noted at first, but after about two weeks, the sleepless rat's paws became ulcerated and they would not heal. The rat who was kept awake soon began to lose weight, even though it had actually eaten more than had the well-rested rat. This weight loss was marked, and was felt to be attributable to the loss of metabolic control (from sleep loss), because both rats exercised the same amount and both had lots of food. The sleepless rat appeared scrawny and dishevelled, and eventually, before the rat died at four weeks of sleeplessness, the animal was extremely wasted – just skin and bones. An autopsy showed only non-specific changes in the animal's brain and tissues, much like those of malnutrition, but it was concluded that prolonged wakefulness was the cause of death.

CAN SLEEP DEPRIVATION CAUSE DEATH IN HUMANS?
Will human beings die if they are kept awake for long enough? Obviously, no one knows for sure, as no humans

Sleep Less, Live Less

The amount you sleep does affect your chances of living longer. Over a period of six years, the American Cancer Society studied one million Americans in San Francisco. Their survival was rated against many lifestyle factors, including sleep patterns. Surprisingly, men who slept four hours a night or less had mortality rates ten times greater than that of those who slept between seven and eight hours! Importantly, those men who overslept, who slept longer than ten hours a night, had double the mortality of those who slept for only seven to eight hours. It seemed that any deviation from the usual sleep requirement for adults of six to eight hours was accompanied by a significant increased risk of mortality. Death from coronary artery disease and strokes was especially prominent in oversleepers. In fact, the National Center for Health Service Research in the United States considers adequate sleep one of the six most important factors affecting illness and death rates; the other lifestyle factors include regular exercise, not smoking, limited consumption of alcohol, regular meal schedules and maintenance of proper weight.

have volunteered to live in a small Plexiglas container with a rotating floor. Many sleep researchers believe that the answer is probably yes, but they agree that it would take a relatively long time, probably weeks, for death to result through this stress alone. Nevertheless, sleep deprivation produces mental and physical changes that are significant threats to health.

Snoring

John was certainly accustomed to being the butt of jokes about his loud snoring; he had endured the kidding and the complaining all his life. Though he himself never heard it, he was well aware of this fault, and grew to be self-conscious and ashamed, even though it was beyond his control. At university, his roommate had to wear earplugs to sleep, and when he imitated John's nighttime snoring and loud whistling to the other students, they laughed uproariously. John laughed too, though he felt humiliated and powerless.

But now, things were different, and the joking was over. John's wife, who was used to his snoring, had noticed changes in her husband that worried her. She was afraid that he might be having some sort of seizure at night, or perhaps – and this was her worst fear – he had developed a brain tumour. How else could she explain his deterioration?

The first change she had noticed was in the snoring itself. Over several months, instead of the regular deep, rattling sound she had grown accustomed to from him, his snoring had developed a more ominous pattern. The regular reverberant, predictable snore would be interrupted by agonizing periods of silence when he wouldn't breathe at all. The change frightened her, and she would often sit up in bed and look over at him. He would be resting comfortably at first, but as the period of silence lengthened, he would begin to move his mouth to try to take a breath, but couldn't seem to take air in. Sometimes he would shake his head or move his hands; he seemed to become more and more agitated the longer the period of silence. Suddenly, with a loud snort and rushing of air, he would be able to breathe again, and would do so several times in a gasping manner. Then he would settle down again, and begin the slow usual snoring. The process would repeat itself again and again.

There were other changes as well. He had recently been diagnosed as having high blood pressure and had been told to lose weight. Though he was only in his early fifties, he had also become impotent, being unable to maintain an erection to ejaculation. He told her he thought the problem was due to 'stress', but she wasn't so sure.

Perhaps because of all these things, his personality had

also changed; she noted that he had become more irritable, less interested in life in general. He had lost some of his *joie de vivre*. His impotence had been a direct blow to his self-confidence, and he was even more ashamed of this problem than he had been about his snoring.

One weekend morning, soon after awakening, he had gone out to get the newspaper and then completely forgotten he had done it. It seemed like such a simple error at the time, but when his wife teased him about it, he became quite agitated. He was adamant that someone else must have placed the newspaper on the kitchen table. In the interest of keeping

---

The Big Snore

Mark Hubbard, who lives in Richmond, British Columbia, holds the record for the loudest snore ever measured. His snore in a sleep laboratory measured an impressive 90 decibels. A decibel is a measure of intensity of sound, and to understand how loud Mark's snoring is, consider that normal human speech is usually in the range of 40 decibels, and that city traffic is usually about 60 to 70 decibels. A jet aeroplane with afterburners registers about 110 decibels, and a pneumatic drill about 120. Each night Mark breaks the Richmond, B.C., traffic bylaw, which restricts traffic sounds to less than 80 decibels. We know from studies in heavy industries that regular exposure to noise above 65 decibels in the workplace can produce hearing loss; earplugs must be worn to prevent damage to hearing. In fact, for habitual snorers of Mark's prowess, hearing loss is fairly common. Anthony Burgess said, 'Laugh and the world laughs with you; snore and you sleep alone.' He may have had Mark in mind!

---

the peace, she backed down and let the incident pass, but she made a doctor's appointment for him. She simply had to know if her worst fears were justified.

SNORING: NO LAUGHING MATTER

'Snoring' is the term used to describe the sound of obstructed breathing during sleep. Though the noise itself may be comical, snoring is no joke, and can in fact be a serious medical problem.

The rattling noise of snoring is caused by vibration of the soft parts of the upper airway. In simple terms, the mouth and throat consist of a bony shell (the vertebrae of the neck, the base of the skull, and the upper and lower jaws), covered on the inside with soft tissues (the muscle of the tongue, and the mucous membrane and muscles that line the back of the mouth and the throat). The hard bony shell of this anatomical region does not change in sleep, but the soft tissues do.

During sleep, the circular muscles at the back of the mouth and the throat relax, and this relaxation allows these soft tissues to be so flaccid that they can vibrate when air passes them. The vibration of these loose soft tissues causes the snoring sound, with its characteristic rumble. There are several different soft-tissue structures that can vibrate in sleep. The tongue, simply a large thick mass of muscle, is attached to the floor of the mouth and the front part of the pharynx. During sleep, when the muscles in this area relax (as is common in deep sleep), the tongue, because of its weight, may passively fall towards the back of the throat. This is more likely to happen if you are lying flat on your back. The movement of the tongue backwards may narrow the airway. Structures at the top of the mouth can also contribute to snoring. Towards the front of the mouth, the roof consists of hard bone – the bony palate – covered with mucous membrane. However, the back third of the roof of the mouth consists only of muscle – the soft (that is, with no bone beneath it) palate. If you open your mouth and look in a mirror, you will see at the back of the roof of your mouth a fold of tissue hanging down in the midline. This is called the uvula, from the Latin *uva*, meaning grape, because early anatomists thought it resembled a small grape hanging down from the soft palate. The uvula functions to direct food away from the space behind the nose and down to the oesophagus below. However, during sleep, this whole area of the muscles of the soft palate, including the grape-like uvula, becomes quite relaxed and sags, obstructing the flow of air. On either side of the uvula lie the tonsils, and below this the pharynx itself, which consists of circular muscle, much like that in the soft palate. All these tissues can relax during deep sleep, and this relaxation, this sagging, has the effect of narrowing the opening through which air must pass. Anything that causes the airway to narrow can cause the sound of noisy, obstructed breathing. In sleep, breathing is regulated through brain centres that initiate respiration by sending a stimulus to the muscle of the diaphragm. This stimulus causes the diaphragm to begin to move; this is the first mechanical step involved in moving air into the chest. As the diaphragm begins to move down, it creates a negative pressure within the lungs themselves, as occurs in opening a bellows. This creation of the negative pressure inside the chest cavity causes air to flow from outside the body through the tubing of the airways, and into the lungs. It's important to understand that this occurs because the movement of the diaphragm, and to a lesser extent the chest wall itself, has created a pressure difference between the air on the outside of the body and the air inside the chest. If there is any obstruction to this air flow (such as that mentioned above), then, as the air does move, it causes vibration of these tissues, and the resulting sound we know as snoring.

In general, about 20 per cent of the adult population snore regularly, with men snoring more than women, and older people snoring more than young people. At age thirty-five, only 20 per cent of men and 5 per cent of women snore. By age sixty though, a full 60 per cent of men and almost 40 per cent of women snore. Snoring is three times more common in people who are overweight than in thin people, and is rated as a serious problem in almost one-third of marriages.

WHY DO WE SNORE?

Anything that causes narrowing of the tubing of the upper airway, or excessive laxity of the tissues that line the airway, causes the air moving past to vibrate, and this vibration of the moving air produces the sound we recognize as snoring. Common causes for snoring include the following:

1. Anything that decreases the tone in the muscles of the upper airway will cause these muscles to be softer, less rigid, and more easily able to vibrate in the moving air. Alcohol is a common offender here, but so are antihistamines, sleeping pills and many other medicines or chemicals that have a sedative or relaxing effect on these tissues.

2. Anything that causes narrowing of the airway anatomically will cause turbulence of the air flowing by, resulting in snoring. In the nose (for in sleep, air is moved through both the mouth and the nose), anatomical obstruction such as nasal polyps, old injuries and old fractures means that the diameter of the tubing through which the air moves is both smaller and irregular. Similarly, swelling of the mucous membranes of the nose (such as might result from allergy or congestion due to a cold) also causes narrowing of the tubing. In the mouth, a large tongue, a short thick neck, or even a receding chin can result in a narrowing of the airway when the muscle support for the tongue is relaxed during deep sleep. On the roof of the mouth, an excessively long soft palate may cause snoring.

3. Obesity causes narrowing of the airway because fat deposits that occur below the mucous membrane of the back of the pharynx produce effective narrowing as well. Hypothyroidism (underactive thyroid) causes the same sort of thickening below this mucous-membrane layer, with the same tendency towards snoring.

4. Any reason for increased amounts of deep sleep will cause increased time for snoring. If you are overtired, chances are you will spend more of the night in deep sleep and, as a result, your chances of snoring are greater.

5. In children, snoring is almost always caused by obstruction to air flow because of enlargement of the tissues of the upper airway. Nasal congestion resulting from allergies or infections (such as colds) is a common cause of snoring. Because the upper airway in children is much smaller than it is in adults, a small amount of congestion or secretion can cause significant snoring. At the back of the throat, snoring is commonly caused by adenoid or tonsil enlargement in children.

Tips for Snorers

1. Lose weight. Striking changes can sometimes be seen in the snoring pattern with the loss of only a few pounds or kilograms.

2. Decrease or stop intake of alcohol, antihistamines, sleeping pills or any other drugs that may be contributing to the problem. All these medicines can cause relaxation of the muscles, and some (namely, alcohol) can cause actual swelling of the tissues. These chemicals can be dangerous; they can convert simple snoring into sleep apnoea (see page 78), with all its problems. Ask your doctor whether any of your prescription medicines may be contributing to the snoring problem.

3. Sleep regularly, and sleep long enough to decrease the amount of deep sleep. The more tired you are, the more deep sleep you will have. Sleep deprivation itself predisposes one to snoring. Regular sleep habits, and adequate time for sleep every night, will help to prevent this tendency.

4. Sleep on your side. Lying on your back narrows the airway more than does lying on your side. Some people pin clothes pegs to the back of their pyjamas, or sew a tennis ball to their pyjamas between the shoulder blades, to make it more comfortable to sleep on their side.

5. Humidify the air that you breathe at night. Dry air causes irritation in the nose and airways and can cause obstruction.

6. Stop smoking and exposing yourself to irritants. Chronic swelling of the mucous membranes from smoking can cause snoring.

7. Raise the head of the bed. This simple manoeuvre often helps to open the airway. A brick placed underneath the legs at the head of the bed is all you need.

8. Anyone who snores significantly should see a doctor for an ear, nose and throat examination (to rule out anatomical or inflammatory causes for narrowing) and for a blood-pressure measurement.

9. Allergies can be the cause of swelling in the nose and throat – either acute or chronic. If you suspect allergy may be a contributing factor, see your doctor.

10. Chronic snoring in children merits medical attention. It can cause decreased performance at school, irritability, inability to concentrate and personality change, all reflections of excessive daytime fatigue.

11. More than three hundred patents have been registered for simple antisnoring devices. Some of the most successful

of these are orthodontic-type devices that hold the airway open. These may be helpful to some people, especially milder cases, are usually inexpensive and have no serious side effects or complications.

12. Surgical treatment for snoring should be a last resort, and usually involves removing the uvula, some of the tissues of the soft palate, and even some of the muscle on the side wall of the pharynx. This can be done by an ear, nose and throat surgeon, using traditional surgical techniques to trim away these tissues or using laser surgery. These surgeries are particularly helpful for those people who have a large redundant uvula or a large soft palate. The success rate in curing snoring approaches 80 per cent but the improvement may be short lived. Like all surgeries, both types involve some complications and are not appropriate for everyone. Consult your doctor.

13. If you suspect that you may have sleep apnoea, and not simple snoring, it is important that you have an adequate medical assessment, preferably a sleep study. Surgery alone rarely cures sleep apnoea.

Tips for Those Who Sleep with Snorers

1. Snorers are usually unaware of their behaviour at night and the sounds that they produce. Because they are asleep (even though it may be only twilight-zone sleep), they cannot hear themselves, so they depend upon you to differentiate mild snoring from obstructive sleep apnoea. Sometimes a tape recording is of value. Remember that at least half of the referrals for obstructive sleep apnoea come from sleep partners. Don't be afraid to initiate evaluation if the snoring is significant, or if there is some evidence of sleep apnoea.

2. Understanding the mechanisms for snoring often leads to lifestyle changes that may help control the problem. Losing weight, stopping alcohol intake and smoking, establishing a regular sleep pattern – all are methods to decrease snoring and in general to promote a healthier lifestyle in your sleeping partner. Insist on these changes.

3. You are entitled to a good night's sleep as well. Normal reactions to having to sleep with someone who snores include such emotions as anger, guilt, disappointment, loneliness and frustration. Chronic fatigue and sleep deprivation are also common. It is not unreasonable to suggest that changes be made in your sleeping arrangements if your bedmate's snoring is bad enough to interfere with your own sleep. Snorers are embarrassed and ashamed about the problem and would rather avoid the issue than face it directly. Snoring is not a personality fault, but it is a problem that you both share. Your insistence on focusing on the problem might very well prevent significant medical complications.

4. As you yourself progress from twilight zone into the deeper layers of sleep, your awareness of the environment decreases. If your sleeping partner's snores disturb you, try to fall asleep first – even if this means going to bed earlier. Some sort of earplug or noise protection is quite appropriate. Many couples who are used to sleeping together find that they don't sleep as well when they sleep alone. However, if your sleeping partner is unable to control snoring to your satisfaction, sleeping in a separate bedroom, even occasionally, may very well relieve some of the chronic fatigue and irritability caused by your sleep deprivation.

Sleep Apnoea

Sleep apnoea is not simply a different kind of snoring. Apnoea comes from the Greek word *apnoia*, meaning without breath, and is the term used to describe repetitive episodes of inability to breathe during sleep. There are two types: obstructive sleep apnoea (caused by an obstruction in the upper airway) and central sleep apnoea (caused by the brain's failure to initiate respiration during sleep).

Studies in a sleep laboratory proved that John, like up to 8 per cent of the adult population, suffered from obstructive sleep apnoea. His episodes of loud snoring, alternating with periods of little or no air flow, were typical. When he was in twilight-zone sleep, he was able to overcome the obstruction to air flow in his upper airway. This milder obstruction produced his regular snoring, which measured 42 decibels. However, as he entered deep sleep, the muscles and tissues in his upper airway became more relaxed. The tissues sagged, the soft palate and uvula lost their tone and the jaw muscles relaxed, allowing his tongue to droop backwards. All these effects caused narrowing of his airway and, as he became more relaxed, eventually the airway closed off completely. When this happened, the respiratory centre in John's brain sent out the signal to his diaphragm to begin the next respiration. The diaphragm contracted, and he began to create a negative pressure within his chest cavity, but it was not enough to overcome the obstruction in his throat. No air moved into his chest. He was, in fact, apnoeic – that is, breathless. Soon, the level of oxygen in his bloodstream began to fall, and his brain began to panic. His heart rate began to rise, as did his blood pressure, sometimes to alarming levels. Eventually his brain would initiate some changes in posture as a nonspecific reaction to the low levels of oxygen. John would move around in bed, perhaps shaking his head or flailing his arms. Eventually, his brain would wake him up to breathe. After being awakened this way, he would enter a lighter stage of sleep, the muscles in his upper airway would regain some of their tone, and he would be able to move air into his chest. The apnoeic spell was over. In the sleep laboratory, these episodes happened to John about three hundred times a night! Basically, when he slept well (that is, when he was in deep sleep), he couldn't breathe. He had a choice: he could either breathe or sleep, but not both together. Only a few seconds after waking up to breathe, he would try to go to sleep again, and the process would repeat itself. No wonder excessive daytime sleepiness is the usual complaint of patients with sleep apnoea. Most patients like John are unaware of the roller-coaster ride between sleep and wakefulness that they take every single night. Though they may have been in bed and thinking they were asleep for some eight to ten hours, many of them actually sleep only a few minutes each night. Some sleep apnoeic patients complain of insomnia; they are simply unable to get back to sleep after the frequent awakenings. Most sleep apnoeic patients seek medical advice because of the observations and complaints of those who sleep with them. Sleep apnoea is usually preceded by several years of snoring, and is uncommon in premenopausal women. The repeated changes in heart rate and blood pressure often lead to chronic hypertension; in fact, if you are a man and you snore, your chance of having high blood pressure doubles. Because the oxygen level in the blood falls regularly during the apnoeic spell, irregular heart rates are very common and can be disastrous. Mark Twain wrote, 'Don't go to sleep – so many people die there.' He may have been thinking of sleep apnoea, because the drop in oxygen in the blood, the high blood pressure, and the irregular heart beat are thought to be a common cause of sudden death in sleep.

Irritability and depression, caused by chronic sleep deprivation, are commonly seen in sleep apnoea. Because people with sleep apnoea enter deep sleep for only a few minutes, they essentially live lives of prolonged sleep deprivation. Automatic behaviour, like John's trip to buy the newspaper, especially soon after awakening, is also common; it simply reflects the chronic, unrefreshing sleep pattern. Because people with sleep apnoea are sleep deprived much of the time, they fall asleep very easily – watching television, during lectures or any time stimulation is minimal. Impotence is common, as is the reflux of acid from the stomach into the back of the oesophagus. This acid is literally sucked up into the chest by the action of the diaphragm creating a negative pressure to try to move air in against the closed upper airway. Sweating at night occurs in almost two-thirds of cases of sleep apnoea. Morning headaches are reported by about 50 per cent.

The rarer form of sleep apnoea, called 'central sleep apnoea', occurs when the brain fails to initiate and coordinate the movements of muscles necessary for respiration. One form of this unusual medical problem has been called 'Ondine's curse', after a maiden in a German legend who punished her former lover by causing him to forget to breathe unless he consciously willed it. The poor man had to actively remember to initiate every single breath for the rest of his life. In contrast to obstructive sleep apnoea, which is far more common, central sleep apnoea does not have the snorting, gurgling respiration that signifies the closure of the airway. It is quite frequent among people with heart disease and should also be reported to your doctor.

TIPS FOR TREATMENT OF SLEEP APNOEA

1. Sleep apnoea can be diagnosed at home or in the sleep laboratory. A simple overnight test recording oxygen levels will pick up most cases. Occasional episodes of apnoea are quite common, and not enough to make the diagnosis. When sleep apnoea is significant there are more than five to ten sleep-apnoea episodes an hour, each lasting longer than 10 seconds. This syndrome puts you at risk for other diseases such as hypertension, heart disease and stroke, and needs to be treated by a physician.

2. All the tips to prevent snoring are applicable to sleep-apnoeic patients (see 'Tips for Snorers', above).

3. If you have sleep apnoea, do not take sleep medicines or sedatives. These chemicals will increase the relaxation in the tissues of the upper airway and make the obstruction worse. In addition, they may very well make your brain less responsive to the low levels of oxygen that the obstruction produces. If your brain does not recognize the falling oxygen level and take steps to remedy it, the consequences could be disastrous. Avoid these medicines – they can be fatal.

4. The most effective treatment for obstructive sleep apnoea is a mask worn at night to keep the airway open. This is called continuous positive airway pressure or CPAP. The CPAP treatment is prescribed by a physician. The mask is attached to the face by straps and then connected to an air pump. It's an ingenious and effective way of treating sleep apnoea. Here's how it works. The main difficulty in obstructive sleep apnoea, as we have seen, is that the tissues of the upper airway tend to collapse and narrow the airway. The mask treatment prevents this collapse because room air is pumped under pressure into the upper airway through the mask, causing these tissues to

remain open. Usually only a small amount of pressure is needed to prevent the tissues collapsing and to stop the obstruction. With this continuous pressure in the mouth, nose, and back of the pharynx, the airway remains open and there is no resistance to air flow when the diaphragm begins its next movement. Patients wear the mask attached to a small pump every night when they sleep. Though it sounds cumbersome, most patients are usually overjoyed with their ability to enter deep sleep again, and to eliminate the chronic sleep deprivation that they have known for years.

4
Insomnia: Can't Get to Sleep, Can't Stay Asleep

Dave was the first to admit that he was obsessive about his sleep. When he awoke each morning, his first thought was to check the time and then figure out the length of his overnight rest. Sleep was so important to him that the calculation of its amount was the barometer of his emotional well-being – it set the tone for his entire day.

Dave had always been a poor sleeper, but the problem worsened suddenly when his father died in a car accident when Dave was only twenty-four. He had been very close to his dad, and the sudden death disturbed the young man greatly, making his own happiness and future seem fragile and pointless. His family doctor took pity on Dave and prescribed nightly diazepam tablets to offer some release from the grief. Dave still remembers the wonderful feeling those first pills gave him – the perfect relaxation from tension, the easing of stress, the fading away of worries and burdens, and the deep restful sleep that followed.

Dave was now a middle-aged salesman, selling insurance

and financial packages to large corporations, and he needed his sleep to be sure he was on his toes. It was a high-pressure job, and his salary depended on his selling abilities, but he had the kind of outgoing, engaging personality that is helpful in jobs requiring personal contact. To outsiders, he seemed energetic and confident, but inside he often wondered if he had chosen the right career, if he would be able to keep up the smiling, confident façade that he presented to the outside world.

Dave found that it was taking more and more of his energy to conduct his meetings. He called them 'his performances' because he saw his role – trying to present his company's financial plans in the best light – as pivotal. He realized that his ability to close a sale rested on the way he handled himself during the meeting and that he must be at his most alert, most dynamic and most engaging.

The nights before his presentations, Dave tried his hardest to get a good night's sleep. He relaxed in a warm bath, then went to bed early and tried to clear his mind of any worries. He lay immobile in his darkened room at ten o'clock, the house quiet, the world still. Then he closed his eyes and tried to go to sleep. It was no use. He would roll over into a different position and try again, forbidding himself to look at the clock. Still sleep would not come. After he had spent an hour or two in this frustrating endeavour, he would rise, wide awake, to go downstairs to get a drink to help him to sleep. Alone in his kitchen, he poured himself a stiff shot or two of alcohol to try to make himself drowsy, but when Dave returned to his bed he was still unable to fall asleep.

The rest of the night was spent in long periods of wakefulness interspersed with very short periods of light sleep. He was awake long before the alarm was due to go off; alert and disgusted with himself, he made espresso coffee, standing once again in his bathrobe in the kitchen. It seemed the more he needed sleep, the less he could depend upon it.

In my office, Dave voiced the complaint of millions of fellow sufferers: 'Why can't I get a decent night's sleep?' He was exasperated and angry; he knew he could be better at his job and at life in general if only he could depend on a restful sleep. 'Tell me, what am I doing wrong?'

The Yin and the Yang of Sleep: Why Insomnia?

Sleep is a normal human phenomenon – a natural and very necessary part of our daily lives. It is so essential that, if denied it, we feel unwell and perform poorly, and eventually, no matter how hard we try, we simply must surrender to its power.

Aristotle, a Greek philosopher who lived three hundred years before Christ, proposed a theory to explain our universal need for sleep. He believed that food, once ingested, released vapours through the process of digestion. These vapours, being warm, rose to the brain and produced the sleepiness that so often follows a heavy meal. After some time, the vapours cooled down, allowing the brain to wake. What he was postulating is that the body produces some sort of chemical that causes sleep. Such a chemical (called a 'hypnotoxin') has for centuries been suspected to be the cause of sleepiness. The substance would be produced in the body by exercise and wakefulness, and when it reached a certain critical level in the brain it would induce sleep. Researchers tried to see if such a chemical existed by taking samples of blood from a sleeping animal and then injecting that blood into an animal who was awake, to see if the injected blood would produce sleep – it wouldn't. Nothing happened. Siamese twins, babies who have not developed in the uterus as separate entities, often share a single organ, such as the liver or the heart, and, though they have the same blood circulation, can have independent sleep–wake schedules – when one of the twins is sleeping, the other may be awake.

These observations imply that there is no single hypnotoxin that causes sleep. The answer is not that simple.

THE SLEEP CENTRE VERSUS THE AWAKE CENTRE

It took a Viennese neurologist to solve the mystery.

Constantine Von Economo was a young volunteer officer in the Austrian Air Force during the First World War, assigned to the medical corps. During the terrible influenza epidemic of those years, he noted that many soldiers infected by the influenza virus were unable to stay awake. Autopsy showed that the virus damaged a specific part of the midbrain, the small bulbous extension of the top of the spinal cord, which lies just at the base of the skull.

Curiously, some of the infected soldiers had exactly the opposite symptom – they couldn't go to sleep at all. Almost all these men died, and autopsy uncovered similar damage in the midbrain with only one difference – those with insomnia always had damage in the back or posterior part of the midbrain, and those who were unable to wake up had damage in the front or anterior part of the same structure. In attempting to explain the conflicting symptoms, Von Economo postulated that two separate centres existed in the brain – one that was responsible for sleep and another, beside the first, that was responsible for wakefulness.

THE WAKE–SLEEP CENTRES

We now understand that there are two distinct centres for

consciousness, both located deep in the base of the brain. One centre controls wakefulness, the other sleeping. Both are active at all times, but their activity varies. With sensory stimulation and signals from the more developed parts of the brain, the wakefulness centre predominates, and the brain 'wakes up'. Sometime later, when sensory stimulation and input from the other parts of the brain decrease, the sleep centre becomes more active and sleep occurs. This duality is common in the human body and is critical in understanding the complexity of sleep. Usually, the alertness centre is dominant, more powerful than the sleeping centre. This makes sense from an evolutionary point of view: because we are vulnerable during sleep, conditions must be just right to allow the weaker sleep centre to take control. The alert centre, which keeps us in our normal waking state and able to defend and protect ourselves, is active most of the time, and relinquishes control to the sleep centre only when conditions are appropriate.

Suppose you haven't slept well the night before, and you have to attend a boring lecture in the afternoon. The hot, stuffy room, the tediously dull topic, the comfortable chair you are sitting in, and the poor sleep you had the night before make chances very good that your sleep centre will become more active and you may begin to nod off. However, in the same comfortable chair, at the same lecture, if you were asked to express an opinion on the boring topic, your wake centre would take over, and all thoughts of sleep would be banished. You would be able to respond to the question, your mind fully alert and reasoning properly. Some minutes later, the two centres may have changed their roles again. It's like a balance of power – one centre simply becomes able to dominate the other for a time.

In general, then, insomnia is a state of imbalance – the

centre for alertness simply overpowers the centre for sleep, preventing the latter from producing the restful effect that is so essential for a peaceful night's sleep.

The alert centre also responds (and this is an important concept for many people who have difficulty sleeping) to the brain's own thought processes, independent of the external environment. Even when you are lying in a darkened, quiet bedroom, where there is very little in the way of external stimulation, the alertness centre can be stimulated by your own thoughts; if they are exciting or worrisome, they can act as stimuli for the awake centre just as effectively as can bright light, sound or other external factors, with the result that sleep is impossible.

The Insomnia Continuum

NORMAL INSOMNIA

Insomnia can be defined as a perception that one's sleep is inadequate, abnormal or unrefreshing. Millions of people have insomnia; a British Sleep Foundation survey in 2000 found that approximately 10 per cent of adults had insomnia.

All these people complained about their sleep, but sometimes not sleeping well can be quite normal. Remember the excitement you used to feel in your childhood, before a holiday or your birthday? Insomnia in children before a special event is normal, a direct result of heightened anticipation. The night before a crucial exam, a job interview, a public-speaking engagement – none of these is usually conducive to quiet, restful, undisturbed sleep. Even falling in love disturbs your sleep, with the flush of exuberance, the self-conscious awareness and the overall sense of well-being all mixed together.

These are all examples of insomnia that is expected and

accepted – in other words, normal. All are part of life's stimulations, and most of them, such as the job interview or falling in love, are positive stimuli – life's good moments – that can result in sleeplessness.

ABNORMAL INSOMNIA

Often, in my role as family doctor in a small town, I am involved with sudden, catastrophic medical events – the death of a child in a car accident, for example – and I am aware that the swift and unexpected tragedy strikes quickly to the very being of the friends and families left behind. They seem barely able to survive the news of the death or accident. They cannot speak, have to sit down, cannot hear, cannot function in the most basic manner as a biological organism – and, of course, they cannot sleep. The blow to their mental state is so devastating that their brain function is thrown into complete disarray, and the alertness centre responds to this stress by absolutely forbidding sleep. Family members and friends request sleeping pills or sedatives to deaden the psychological pain, but we recognize that this kind of reaction to personal calamity is expected and usual; it is, in fact, the normal response to an abnormal situation. The insomnia that results is just as predictable and universal as the anguish itself, and is all part of the brain's way of coping with the idea of a new world without the loved one.

CHRONIC INSOMNIA

Sometimes, however, our sleep is difficult for reasons other than joyful anticipation or reaction to calamity. Sometimes, without any obvious cause, we lie awake for hours trying to sleep – and sleep simply will not come. Sometimes it does come, but then is broken again and again, each awakening documented by the fluorescent numbers on a digital clock mocking our efforts to rest. Sometimes the alertness centre dominates all night long, preventing the weaker sleep centre from exerting its influence over the brain and body, and the war goes on all night. Eventually, next morning, the alert centre emerges the victor, and we rise unrefreshed from the battlefield to begin another exhausting day. This chronic insomnia can be classified into three different types: difficulty in getting to sleep, difficulty in staying asleep (particularly with repeated awakenings), and too short a sleep to be restful (waking up too early). Each of these sleep problems has its own causes, and an understanding of them allows us to adopt an approach to treating the disturbed sleep pattern.

Can't Get to Sleep

One of the commonest forms of insomnia is that frustrating inability to drift off to sleep. We use the phrase 'falling asleep' to describe the process of entering the altered level of consciousness of the first stages of sleep – twilight zone – and this image of 'falling' is significant. It describes the light, gentle, floating sensation so common in the early part of sleep, a kind of drifting, often described as being a lowering or a light feeling of falling, a descent away from the awake state. We know from electroencephalograms recorded in the sleep laboratory that the moment of sleep occurs quite suddenly and is specific, but the feeling of restful serenity that precedes it does not have its own EEG rhythm – it looks just like waking life. Normally it takes up to twenty minutes for most people to fall asleep, a period called 'sleep latency', and anything over thirty minutes is abnormal. Many good sleepers can fall asleep in two minutes or less, 'as soon as the head hits the pillow', but many insomniacs lie with their eyes resolutely closed for hours, yet sleep will not come. There are many reasons why, but all of them involve over-activity of the alert or awakeness centre.

THE PRECONDITIONS OF SLEEP

Sleep is often impossible without certain preconditions being met. We have all been in the situation where the room was far too hot, or the noise from the hotel room next door was just too loud, or the sofa was simply too uncomfortable to allow us to drift off. Remember, the alertness centre is acti-vated by external stimuli, so sleeping on a bed of nails like a Hindu fakir is impossible for most of us – the sleep centre is simply overpowered by the sensation of pain. We need a reasonable set of physical preconditions or sleep will not come.

First, we need to be tired. It is much more difficult to fall asleep when the normal circadian rhythm is at its peak, and much easier when the rhythm is at a trough (in midafter-noon or in the wee hours of the morning). If we are well rested, we are less tired, and less likely to be able to drift off.

Second, we need a reasonable room temperature. Sleep is virtually impossible above 100°F (38°C), and in general the optimal temperature for sleep is between 64° and 72°F (18° and 22°C). The best temperature for sleep varies fairly widely from person to person and it is rarely shared by a couple. Generally, men are warmer than women while sleeping, and thus require fewer blankets, a lower setting on the electric blanket, fewer bedclothes, and more skin exposed (which is why many men stick their feet out from underneath the covers at the end of the bed).

Third, we need a reasonably soft yet supportive structure

beneath us. The modern mattress allows us a much better sleep than our ancestors enjoyed, though there seems little difference among the various types of mattresses available. Despite claims to the contrary, waterbeds produce no significant change in sleep patterns, although individual people may see a difference. We also prefer to be flat when sleeping – horizontal, instead of sitting upright. Though it is possible to fall asleep while sitting if you're tired enough, the sleep you get is not as refreshing and is shorter, with more frequent awakenings. Similarly, sleeping on a hard surface, such as a hardwood floor, produces the same kind of reduction of quality in sleep.

We also need quiet – remember, the alert centre responds to external stimuli – though there are some paradoxes here. The deeper the sleep, the louder the noise needed to wake you, but there's more to it than that. Noises that have some connotation for you, such as the whimper of an infant, are much more likely to wake you up than are some other emotionally neutral noises of the same intensity – traffic noise, for example. Before we fall asleep, absolute quiet is not needed; in fact, some people are able to fall asleep faster when non-specific or 'white' noise is audible in the background. (Bedroom appliances that produce white noise are commercially available.) The regularity, the predictability of the sound seems to be the significant aspect, not the type of noise. Sudden, unpredictable changes in pitch and volume prevent sleep much more dramatically than do low, drone-type noises, which often encourage it. Women are more sensitive to sound than are men, and sensitivity to sound increases with age – the elderly are more easily awakened by lighter sounds.

We seem to be able to tolerate some horrendous noises, such as snoring, if we ourselves make them. There is nothing more frustrating than lying awake listening to your bed partner snore, and having that sound prevent your drifting off to sleep. However, though the snore will prevent you from entering sleep, many people find that it will not awaken them – and they know that their sleep will be much more refreshing if they are able to fall asleep before the snoring bed partner.

YOU CAN'T FORCE YOURSELF TO GO TO SLEEP

Last, and this is probably one of the most difficult pre-conditions of sleep, we need to be calm, relaxed and serene. We need to be able to turn down the dominance of the alertness centre to allow the weaker sleep centre to take over. It is important to realize that we can't force the sleep centre to dominate – there is nothing we can do to make ourselves sleepier, in other words; we simply have to learn to decrease the activity of the alertness centre, to make ourselves less awake, less alert. The process of going to sleep is an active one, but the action is all directed towards minimizing the power of the alertness centre, not increasing the power of the sleep centre. For example, many insomniacs try too hard to fall asleep. They lie in their beds, eyes tightly closed, teeth clenched, and focus their thoughts on getting to sleep. They convince themselves that the next few minutes will be crucial in getting a good night's sleep and to their performance the next day. Then they imagine what it will be like if they haven't been able to sleep well – that awful draggy feeling, the headache, the irritability – and anticipate the frustration of knowing that they will not be their best.

The problem is that these sleepers are trying too hard to fall asleep. The cerebral activity of willing sleep to come, of considering the awful consequences of failure, of self-doubt and anger – all function to stimulate the alertness centre, to increase its activity and thus completely dominate the brain's function. The very act of trying so hard effectively banishes any hope of sleep. Actively willing sleep to come doesn't work; they need to learn to allow sleep to come by decreasing the power of the awake centre.

Most people find that it is impossible to easily drop off to sleep unless they have brushed their teeth. The physical act of using toothpaste and brush to polish up the teeth has little effect on sleep, but most of us have learned that this daily task of hygiene is best fitted into the day at this particular time. We have learned from a young age that regular brushing of the teeth is a *good thing*, and we have come to associate that brushing with bedtime. In effect, we are 'conditioned' to associate the ritual of preparing for bed with sleep.

Ivan Pavlov (1849–1936), a Russian physiologist, conducted a famous set of experiments that showed that conditioning was an important biological phenomenon. In his laboratory, he kept a group of dogs to whom he fed huge chunks of succulent meat only once per day. Just before he fed them, he rang a bell for several seconds. The bell sounded, then the food arrived, and the animals dug in, wolfing down their meat. After a while, Pavlov began to lengthen the time between the bell and the actual arrival of the meat. Eventually, he simply rang the bell – no meat was offered – and when he rang it, the dogs began to anticipate the food. They would pace back and forth in their cages, with huge wet globs of saliva flowing out of their mouths. The important point was that the dogs learned to associate the bell with the food, and sounding the bell began to produce the physiological changes that were associated with feeding. This phenomenon Pavlov called a 'conditioned reflex', the change in physiology that was associated with the stimulus of the bell.

The concept is very important for insomnia – it's the reason you can't easily fall asleep without brushing your teeth. For years, we have associated brushing our teeth – the clean feeling of newly polished teeth, the fresh taste of toothpaste, the remembered approval we received for this single act of self-care – with the calm before sleep. Brushing our teeth is our bell, and we need to ring it before we can decrease the activity of the waking centre. Some people must check that their home is secure and have difficulty sleeping with the doors unlocked. For some, checking the children is another precondition; for others, reading a chapter or two or perhaps cuddling with their bed partner has the same function. The particular 'bells' may be different, but we all seem to have them.

One of my patients reported to me that he had a great deal of trouble falling asleep every night in his suburban bedroom and often tossed and turned for an hour or so before sleep would finally come. However, at his cottage on a lake, he dropped off to sleep so easily that he couldn't even read in bed. It wasn't the difference in the bed or the room. The release of stress and anxiety associated with his stay at the cottage was the factor – he slept just as easily while out backpacking, even while lying in a sleeping bag in his tent in the middle of a downpour!

If you sleep better somewhere other than in your own bed, this may mean that the bed and the bedroom have connotations that are keeping you up. Perhaps you have learned to dislike intensely the futile feeling of wanting sleep to come, or perhaps you know that, as soon as you lie down, the pressure is once again on you to fall asleep.

Perhaps the bed is a site for conflict with your partner –

not open warfare, but a smouldering misunderstanding about sleep or sex or some other aspect of your relationship. Perhaps the frustration of trying so hard to sleep without success is associated with this particular room, this bed, this digital clock with its disturbing alarm.

You may be reacting like the dogs in Pavlov's laboratory.

In the same vein, many insomniacs are easily able to drift off in the den watching television after dinner, but then lie wide awake for the rest of the night in bed. Because insomniacs are always tired, all day every day, they find themselves among the first to begin to nod during the after-lunch lecture – sleep seems so easy, so imperative it cannot be denied, yet night sleep will not come on demand. Some of these patterns may be related to the associations the bedroom has for you – the worry you engage in there as well as the exertion of trying to fall asleep (as opposed to simply letting sleep come).

Sleep and the Alertness Dimmer Switch

The alertness centre cannot suddenly be switched off, just because you decide it's time to get into bed and go to sleep. It's rather like a dimmer switch for an overhead light – turning it one way gradually increases the amount of light, and turning it the other way gradually decreases the amount of light. Alertness isn't controlled by a simple on–off switch, as most lamps are; it's a gradual process of decrease in power that allows the sleep centre to take control.

This concept of gradually 'dimming' your alertness and awareness of the outside world and its problems is quite essential – you can't fall asleep without it. Many of the rituals, the simple acts that precede sleep, are part of this dimming process.

HOW TO TELL IF YOU ARE OVERALERT

Excessive activity of the alertness centre is usually easily identified; it commonly produces a whole set of symptoms, though not all are present in every case. Increased muscle tension is often a symptom, specifically in the muscles of the neck (producing headache or neckache), the muscles of the jaw (producing pain on the side of the head in the temple area, or pain in the ear or the jaw itself), and the muscles of the back (producing pain and stiffness in this area). Another sign of an overactive alertness centre is the excess energy syndrome – the inability to sit still, as indicated by the constant tapping of toes and drumming of fingers or other types of fidgeting. In these situations, the muscles are overstimulated, in a perpetual state of 'red alert', prepared to act quickly in response to any change or threat. This muscular reaction is part of our generalized response to stress, and is something we share with most other animals. Stress causes increased awareness of the external environment, and prepares us for either a fight or flight response – which means our muscles had better be ready for immediate action. If you are under stress all day long (and who among us is not?), your muscles are simply reacting to this. They are prepared for a sudden move – excitable and ready to function. In this state of readiness for action, you may notice that your heart is pounding, your hands and feet are cool and your whole body is ready to pounce. These effects, all part of the general arousal state, are quite appropriate if you are being threatened – say, by an attacking wild animal – but they are completely incompatible with sleep. Unfortunately, for many of us, the stresses of everyday life have produced a reaction of this type that lasts, not for a moment or two when we are threatened, but for the entire twenty-four-hour day. This abnormal stress response guarantees that we will have trouble sleeping.

In addition to these physical signs of excess stress, its psychological signs are fairly easy to identify – you can't relax and can't stop your mind from racing from thought to thought and from worry to worry. Often these racing thoughts are preceded by the phrase 'What if?' – a sign of anxiety. Some anxiety is a useful survival tool; it helps us to plan strategies for the future as the mind analyzes the different possibilities and our reactions to them, but too much anxiety soon results in overstimulation, with the emotional context of the worry, the anguish, far outweighing any benefits of the planned response. If you cannot slow your thoughts down before going to sleep, you will not be able to dim the alertness centre to allow sleep to come.

How to Turn Down Your Alertness Centre

Some of us have no trouble falling asleep, taking as little as one to two minutes to enter twilight-zone sleep. As is the case for all human functions, there is quite a bit of variation among us as to our capacity to sleep. Some are simply better at it than others, being able to dim their arousal switches with annoying ease and have their sleep centre dominate within minutes.

Champion sleepers – just like brilliant singers or graceful basketball players – have an innate ability that makes them better at it than most other people. The rest of us mere mortals need to work at dimming our alertness centres, or singing, or playing basketball.

Look carefully at your routine in the evening. Do you race around like the proverbial headless chicken and then flop into bed expecting sleep to come? If so, try to organize your day so that the last part of it does not involve stimulating mental activity. Is the late-evening discussion with your teenage daughter about homework contributing to your increased arousal state? Are you so anxious about getting your infant to sleep that your concern, paradoxically, prevents *you* from sleeping? Exercise helps to alleviate some of the stress that prevents sleep, but not if it is done right before you go to bed. Your evening jog should be at least two to three hours before bedtime; otherwise your poor body won't know whether it should be pumped up or deflated. Many insomniacs fill the time they spend waiting for sleep with a review of upcoming events, and this often leads to anticipation of problems or conflicts. In short, they worry about tomorrow (or yesterday) while worrying whether or not they can get to sleep. 'Worry,' wrote Anglican scholar William Ralph Inge, 'is interest paid on trouble before it falls due.'

At bedtime, try to clear your mind of this kind of arousing material. Some psychiatrists go so far as to suggest that you establish a 'worry time', a specific half-hour or so after supper where this kind of planning or rehashing is done. It works like this: set aside 20 or 30 minutes each evening for worry – 'planning' is perhaps a more positive description of the activity – and then use this time to examine anticipated problems in detail. Begin by writing down the problem – say, a concern about your sister's marriage, or your son's difficulty with maths, or a financial worry – and then write down the probable solutions or approaches, including their benefits and complications.

Many worries are nonspecific gut reactions, emotional responses to perceived problems, and they take a lot of your energy. Because they are mainly emotional, they are difficult to pin down, but when you force yourself to actually write them down in detail, strange things happen – you literally define the problem in your mind, give it a name, and limit it by writing down its specific aspects. By doing so, you have made the problem finite – it has an edge, a boundary, instead of being a free-floating amorphous fear or concern. Once the problem has a definite boundary, you can begin to examine it, turning it over and looking at all sides, at all facets, and examining it closely from different angles to uncover its complications and possible solutions. Most of these sorts of worries don't have a simple answer; if they did, we would have dismissed them long ago. But even frustrating problems, those not easily solved, can be defined. This can be accomplished by simply talking about the problem, but the act of writing it down leads to the specific thoughtful detail that makes the solution easier to imagine.

Many problems are not easy to face. It can be difficult to find a solution for such concerns as the feeling that you have not accomplished what you set out to in life, or the sense of worthlessness that so many older people experience, or the pain when your love is not returned by your mate or child. By arranging a regularly scheduled time to work on these concerns, you can free your mind during the time you're lying in bed waiting for sleep to come, relax and turn down your alertness centre.

Relaxation Is the Key

If relaxation, the release from intense concentration on day-to-day worries, is essential for sleep, how can we achieve it?

There are many methods of achieving relaxation, of disengaging your mind from the concerns of the day, that will allow you to sleep. Counting sheep, for example, is a boring, repetitive, nonproductive task, and all those qualities help decrease arousal. While counting, your mind focuses on the numbers themselves, as you visualize a purposeless, non-threatening scene – namely, the sheep parading past you. You can focus your mind on other neutral images, such as counting slowly from one hundred down to zero, and visualizing the numbers as you count, with the same effect.

Remembering a restful scene to try to recapture the feeling of peace associated with it is also very helpful. Imagine yourself in a pleasant situation from your past – for example, on vacation, lying on a beach in the warm summer sun. Focus on the relaxation, the lack of tension in your muscles as you lie still, feel the warm sun on your skin, smell the water nearby and listen to the soft lapping of the waves. By focusing on each of the senses in turn, you can create the overall serene feeling of relaxation.

Meditation of any kind will achieve the same effect. It's fairly easy to learn, and quite relaxing. Once you have mastered the technique, it can be used to manage stress at any time of the day or night. It is particularly helpful for those people who have difficulty getting to sleep or who awaken frequently and have difficulty returning to sleep.

Counteracting the increased muscle tension associated with stress is also helpful. A hot bath taken sometime before sleep allows the tight muscles to relax, and simple stretching exercises also work. These decrease the tension associated with excessive alertness, and are soothing in themselves. Exercises before bed often help prevent leg cramps as well. Massage similarly relaxes muscles. One of my patients falls asleep in seconds when his bald head is massaged, but tosses and turns for forty-five minutes if it is not!

Regular Sleep Schedules and Napping

It is essential to try to keep your wake-up time constant –

even on weekends. Try to impose a schedule on your sleep–wake cycle; the more predictable and regular that schedule is, the better you adapt to it, and the better you sleep. If you try on some mornings to sleep in, to catch up on sleep you might have missed, you'll simply find it more difficult to fall asleep that night and wake up the next day at the same time. Remember, your circadian rhythm is longer than twenty-four hours and must be reset each morning. For this reason, avoid late nights and irregular bedtimes. If you keep a record of your sleep, a sleep log, you will often see marked variations – for example, late-night parties or other activities mixed in with more reasonable bedtimes. Such variation confuses your sleep–wake cycle; a predictable pattern helps sleep come more easily as your body and brain anticipate the diminished arousal that is so necessary for sleep to begin. Similarly, you should refrain from consuming caffeine and alcohol, or at least minimize your intake.

For insomniacs, the short nap is usually counterproductive. If you achieve some of your well-deserved rest by napping in the afternoon, chances are you will be less likely to sleep well that night, especially if the nap was quite refreshing. Some people, especially seniors, are able to fit a short nap into their schedule (Winston Churchill did almost every day), but most insomniacs simply compound the problem by trying to sleep at other times.

Believe it or not, many insomniacs spend too much time in bed. Because it might take a long time to fall asleep, and because their sleep is so unrefreshing, it's not uncommon for insomniacs to spend eight to twelve hours in bed every day! Unfortunately, this behaviour perpetuates the connotation of frustration and anger the bedroom comes to have. Insomniacs spend that much time in bed because it takes them an hour to fall asleep; they awaken many times during the night, and, in general, their sleep is not refreshing so they need more of it to get the same feeling of rest.

Try to spend just as much time in bed as you used to before your insomnia – on average, eight hours is plenty. Spending longer may actually be contributing to the problem, as we know that deep, refreshing sleep occurs early in the night for most tired sleepers. You may be spending all night in superficial twilight-zone–type sleep instead of the usual pattern of restorative sleep, simply because that's what your body has learned to do.

Is Your Insomnia a Psychological Symptom?

Insomnia is not a disease; it is simply a symptom, a complaint caused by altered body function. As is true for all symptoms, the specific reason for it must be sought. Sometimes insomnia is a symptom of psychological or emotional problems, particularly depression or excess anxiety, and to alleviate the symptom, you must address the underlying problem. Of those people who see a sleep specialist with a complaint of chronic insomnia (insomnia that has lasted for at least three months), almost 50 per cent have some kind of emotional or psychological problem as the underlying cause of poor sleep.

ARE YOU DEPRESSED?
Severe clinical depression is almost always accompanied by some kind of sleep disorder. This association is so strong that depression is rarely the diagnosis if the patient's sleep is unchanged. Classically, the most common change in sleep pattern in depression is that of early-morning awakening – that is, sleep that ends significantly earlier than usual, perhaps

at four or five o'clock instead of at six or seven o'clock – and an inability to return to sleep. Other common sleep abnormalities in depression include difficulty in falling asleep, and repeated awakenings. Not all depressed patients have shortened, unrefreshing sleep though; some 15 per cent are excessively drowsy and sleep far too much. In the sleep laboratory, depressed patients have their first REM segment earlier in the night and experience a decrease in deep sleep, an increase in arousals, and sleep that is lighter, shorter and more disturbed.

Depression is essentially a change in the way you feel, and

Are You Depressed?

Depression is a common cause of chronic insomnia, particularly insomnia that does not respond to simple treatments. Here is a list of the common symptoms and signs of depression.

1. Depressed mood – a sense of sadness or melancholy, a tendency to interpret things in a negative way, a sense of worthlessness or gloom, present most of the day, nearly every day.
2. Markedly diminished interest or pleasure in all, or almost all, activities of the day, nearly every day.
3. Significant weight loss or weight gain not attributable to change in diet.
4. Significant change in sleep pattern – either insomnia (early-morning awakenings, difficulty in sleeping or repeated awakenings), or excessive sleep.
5. Fatigue or loss of energy – a feeling of tiredness, of not having the strength to go on.
6. Feelings of worthlessness or excessive or inappropriate guilt, nearly every day.
7. Diminished ability to think or concentrate – an indecisiveness or difficulty in making decisions, or in concentrating in general.
8. Recurring thoughts of death, or thoughts of what the world would be like without you.

Depression is not your fault. It is not something that you have caused, nor does it reflect weakness of character. It is usually a treatable medical problem, and appropriate treatment usually enriches your life substantially. See your doctor.

it always brings with it sadness or a sense of hopelessness, a loss of enjoyment of life, as well as fatigue. Changes in weight (most patients lose weight) and decrease in appetite are very common, as is withdrawal from social interactions with other people. A lack of enjoyment in things that used to give you pleasure, and an overwhelming sense of purposelessness, or even hopelessness with thoughts of suicide, are common.

Ten per cent of men and twenty per cent of women will suffer some sort of depression in their lives, either bipolar mood disorder (a mixture of extreme highs and lows) or a major unipolar (unrelieved low) depression.

Being depressed does not mean that you are crazy or psychotic. Depression is simply a continuum of human response ranging from a very mild sense of melancholy or dissatisfaction to a severe, overwhelming blackness. The point is that, if depression is causing your insomnia, finding help for the depression will make your sleep, and your life, better. Many depressed people will not admit that they have a problem, seeing it as some sort of weakness in their moral fibre; they struggle on for years, sometimes much of their lives, without letting their feelings out. This so-called hidden depression is commonly a reason for sleep difficulties, as well as for a pervasive loss of enjoyment in their lives. Though the treatment of depression is rarely simple, these people often find that attention to the problem makes a dramatic difference in their feeling of well-being, their interactions with their friends and families, their self-esteem, and their symptoms, including insomnia. Treatment often allows such people, for the first time in years, to once again take pleasure in life.

ANXIETY AS A CAUSE OF INSOMNIA

If you have difficulty getting to sleep and also experience a persistent feeling of uneasiness throughout the day, you may very well have one of the psychological diseases called the 'anxiety disorders'. We all have some anxiety; it's the state of being uneasy, apprehensive or worried about what may happen. It's a normal human emotion, and we all have it when we must take a driving test or some other examination, or give a short speech of introduction at a meeting. But for most of us anxiety is a temporary phenomenon that occurs before a stressful situation and disappears when it is over. However, for some, excessive persisting anxiety is a powerful destructive force, robbing life of much of its pleasure. It can be present all the time, not just intermittently, and when a vague fear or tension is with us day and night it prevents relaxation and leads to fussing and fretting over the simplest decisions, and paralyzed inaction resulting from apprehension of what might occur. Anxiety itself is an unpleasant feeling of fear and agitation arising when the mind considers what may occur in the future. If it is present all the time, psychologists refer to it as 'generalized anxiety disorder'. A second common pattern of abnormal anxiety is 'panic disorder', in which a sudden, intense, frightening wave of anxiety or panic occurs without warning. These episodes of anxiety are so severe that they usually produce physical symptoms as well as emotional ones – people suddenly become nauseated and feel dizzy, their chests are tight, their hearts are racing, they are short of breath, they break out in a sweat, and often have abdominal pain and severe headache. These disturbing, unpredictable episodes of acute anxiety are, of course, extremely frightening. Patients often go to a hospital casualty department, believing that they have had a heart attack, a stroke or other life-threatening medical emergency. Anxiety may also reveal itself in the pattern of 'phobias' –

Do You Suffer from Excessive Anxiety?

Anxiety is the unpleasant feeling of fear or apprehension about what might occur in the future. It is a normal human emotion, which often helps us prepare for the future by considering various possibilities, but signs of excessive anxiety include the following:

1. Unrealistic or excessive worry or apprehension about life's circumstances, particularly when these worries are out of proportion to the problem – for example, worrying about possible misfortune to a child who is in no danger.

2. A feeling of being keyed-up or on edge, of being 'hyper' or overly sensitive to changes in the environment, such as the telephone ringing or other noise. A feeling of being unable to relax.

3. A difficulty in concentrating or 'mind going blank' because of worry; a constant feeling of being rushed.

4. Irritability, associated with fatigue.

5. Trouble falling asleep or staying asleep.

6. Excessive trembling, twitching or a feeling of being shaky in the muscles; increased muscle tension, aches or soreness, and susceptibility to fatigue.

7. Recurring episodes of shortness of breath, smothering sensations, palpitations, sweating or cold clammy hands, dry mouth, dizziness, nausea, diarrhoea or other abdominal distress, associated with an intense fear or worry that something terrible is about to happen. These symptoms may occur at night and wake you from sleep.

8. A persisting feeling of being 'out of control', 'ready to burst inside', inability to cope, etc.

Many of the symptoms of anxiety can be caused by other medical disorders (such as hyperthyroidism) or excessive use of caffeine or other stimulants. Anxiety disorders, like depression, are well-recognized medical problems; they are not indications of weakness or other personal faults. Attention to treatment often allows patients the ability to once again take control of their emotions, and to take pleasure in life.

---

severe, unwarranted, illogical fears associated with objects or activities – or in 'obsessive-compulsive disorder', where an overwhelming need to perform repetitive, unnecessary tasks dominates over reason. Though they know it is not appropriate, or logical, these patients are compelled to do repetitive, often symbolic tasks (such as washing the hands), and are driven by a deep-seated fear of the consequences of not doing so. One of the most dramatic forms of anxiety is 'post-traumatic stress disorder', a severe and often disabling form of stress associated with a previous horrendous experience, such as the atrocities of war, violent crime or disaster.

All these anxieties can cause difficulty with sleep. About 25 per cent of patients seen by sleep specialists are found to have excessive anxiety. In general, the cardinal effect of anxiety on sleep is that it delays onset – the anxiety state prevents dimming of the alertness centre, and, even if sleep does come, frequent awakenings throughout the night, with a shorter, lighter, less refreshing sleep, usually follow. Anxiety takes a lot of energy, and this use of energy, in combination with the poor, unrefreshing sleep, causes these patients to be tired all day long.

Can't Stay Asleep

One common pattern of insomnia involves awakening and having difficulty returning to sleep. We all rise from sleep to the awake state every night an average of ten to fifteen times, but most of us are able to simply shift position, adjust the covers and quickly head back down into restful sleep. We're not even aware in many cases that we awoke at all. For some people these short, brief arousals are not simply a part of their cycle of sleep but rather interrupt the sleep completely. These people awaken, and very quickly become fully alert (even if they leave their eyes closed), and cannot return to sleep, no matter what they do. Eventually they look at the clock and their worst fears are realized – it's three or four or five o'clock in the morning, and they know that sleep will not come again to them that night. They lie in bed trying to force sleep to return, and, when they finally give up, they rise unrefreshed in the early dawn. Others are able to return to sleep, but only after a prolonged period of alertness; they, too, are unable to obtain their much-needed rest in bed.

What seems to be happening in both cases is that the alertness centre has become dominant very quickly, preventing the sleep centre from controlling brain function.

Normal sleepers have a rhythm to their sleep – a fairly regular rising and then falling in level of consciousness and depth of sleep. They rise from a deep sleep all the way to a brief arousal, but then quickly they descend again to the next phase. The change to arousal is simply part of the cycle, the way the peak of an ocean wave is followed by a trough and then the next peak. Those who awaken frequently are different – their sleep cycle is interrupted each time they rise to this level of arousal. It's as if they have to try to begin to go to sleep ten to fifteen times a night, in addition to the first time! Instead of being one continuous flow, with different levels of alertness, their sleep is broken into short, separate periods of rest, each in turn interrupted by periods of being fully awake. It's a very frustrating, unrefreshing pattern, night after night.

WHY ARE YOU AWAKENING?
Sometimes there is a very good reason for you to awaken fully in the night. A distended bladder from the cup of tea that you had after supper, the arthritis pain in your back, the heat of the electric blanket that you forgot to turn off, the heartburn caused by the late-night snack – all are good reasons for awakening. Those who suffer from frequent

awakenings should look carefully at the pattern of their interrupted sleep to see if there is a good reason for these to occur. Can you change your schedule to allow you to sleep restfully? For many older people, distention of the bladder is a common reason for disturbed sleep with frequent awakenings, and attention to this problem often solves the sleep disruption. Similarly, anything that produces superficial sleep will cause more frequent awakenings. Perhaps caffeine intake during the day, or even exposure to nicotine from secondhand smoke, may be causing a more superficial sleep, and thus predisposing you to more frequent awakenings. In addition to examining the reasons for awakening, or the reasons for a superficial sleep that is easily disrupted, attention to the physical details of the sleeping environment is important. Do you wake up because you are cold, or because the noises of the street are different, or because the loud snoring of your bed partner is causing the awakening?

There are some people, though, who even after examination of these causes of frequent awakenings seem to find themselves awake for no good reason several times throughout the night. Those who can find no reason why they awaken simply have to deal with the awakenings when they occur.

The secret is to consider that each of these awakenings essentially means that sleep has been completely interrupted and that you must try to go to sleep again. Each of these episodes is essentially a recreation of the situation when you first tried to go to sleep at the beginning of the night. Therefore, you must simply try to go to sleep again, using the same techniques that allowed you to ease into sleep earlier. Use the tricks of disengaging your mind from the worries of the day, relax the muscles of your body, and focus on dimming the alertness centre so that the sleep centre might once again take over. Being awake in the middle of the night is very frustrating, particularly if it occurs regularly, and you must not let the frustration build by lying in bed, forcefully trying to make sleep come. If you are unable to fall asleep within ten or fifteen minutes, it is quite appropriate to leave the bed and move to another room, where you can begin the process of falling asleep again – perhaps reading a book, doing simple stretching exercises, listening to music or engaging in some other activity that allows the alertness centre to relinquish its domination.

Sleep and Its Environment

Besides the interior factor of your particular sleep–awake cycle, various aspects of the exterior environment can have an effect on your ability to fall asleep and stay asleep.

NOISE AND SLEEP
Most people underestimate the effect of noise, or lack of it, on their sleep. We all know how annoying it is to hear the dripping of a tap in another room, or the clock ticking away in the silence of the night, but some of us cannot sleep without some sort of background noise – for example, the radio playing softly or the low hum of a fan or air conditioner.

The amount of noise that we can tolerate during sleep varies tremendously from one person to another. Some people are awakened by a light 15-decibel whimper, while others can sleep soundly through noises as loud as 100 decibels, a noise level comparable to that in an all-night disco bar. Generally, much less noise is needed to awaken you in twilight-zone sleep than in deep sleep, and you are more likely to be roused by noise in the first part or in the last part of sleep, since you are more aware of changes in your environment during those stages of the sleep cycle. Interestingly, less sound is needed to awaken someone if the sound is a recognizable, meaningful one, rather than a non-specific, generic sound. Women are awakened more easily than men by a sudden noise, and young people sleep through more noise than do their seniors, who are more easily awakened by minor disturbances. A noise loud enough to waken a seventy-year-old will cause only a shift into twilight-zone sleep for most twenty-five-year-old sleepers.

It makes good evolutionary sense that sudden, unexpected noise alarms or awakens us. Remember, we are very vulnerable in sleep, so we need to be able to awaken in response to any noise that might signify danger. On the one hand, a sudden noise is more likely to be a threat to us, a source of harm, than a gentle, comforting sound.

On the other hand, soft, steady rhythmic noise is often helpful in falling asleep. Bach's *Goldberg Variations* are tender and quiet piano solos written at the request of a prince who wanted some music to help him sleep. However, some people would find that listening to piano music would forbid sleep. The point is, there is quite a bit of individual variation, and you should experiment to see what works for you. Earplugs can be a help for those who seem to be aware of every little noise, and some low background sound, such as a fan running on low speed, may help muffle the faint irregular sounds the house makes as you try to rest. This effect is called 'blocking' and it works for many people. Sometimes, such as when a dripping tap captures your full attention, your hearing actually becomes more acute while you are trying to go to sleep and you pick up sounds that you would normally not hear. This seeming paradox can be explained in part by the fact that the sounds you make during normal activity cease when you are trying to drop off to sleep, and the relative silence amplifies what little sound there is. Some soft, soothing, regular background noise in this situation is very helpful.

THE PRINCESS AND THE PEA
In this famous fairy tale, the princess was so sensitive, so tender-skinned, that she was able to feel a small pea placed beneath mattresses stacked, one on one, to the sky, every time she tried to go to sleep.

It's true that, for some people, the specifics of the bed and the mattress are very important. However, the variety of personal preferences makes it hard to generalize. Some people prefer a soft mattress, but most people sleep better on a firm one that is not lumpy and does not sag in the middle. It is prudent to inspect your bed and mattress for wear and tear, and you might want to try to sleep with the mattress directly on the floor one night, as this gives it better support. Beds don't last forever, and mattresses usually need replacing at least every seven to ten years.

Sleep Position: Does How You Sleep Affect How Well You Sleep?

In an average night, most sleepers change position twenty to forty times, and remain in a particular position for an average of fifteen minutes. In addition, we all have a repertoire of positions – those that we seem to like best – and we usually use them night after night. Poor sleepers generally turn or change position much more frequently during the night than do good sleepers, though all sleepers must adjust

Pillow Talk

Ideally, your pillow should allow your head to rest in a neutral position, with the neck straight. If you lie on your back and sleep with two pillows, your neck will be flexed throughout much of the night, and, during dream sleep, when the muscles in your neck relax, the ligaments are the only thing holding the neck in that position and they will be stretched for several hours. As a result, your neck will be sore in the morning. Similarly, if you sleep on your side and you have a single, thin pillow, your neck might very well be tilted towards the side you are sleeping on all night. This compresses the small joints on that side of the neck, and conversely stretches open the small joints on the other side of the neck. If your neck is sore every morning when you awake, the position of your neck throughout the night probably has caused the problem. The neck should be maintained in a straight line, just as it is when you are standing erect, without being flexed (as it is when your chin rests on your chest) or extended (as it is when you look up towards the sky). Pillows often trigger allergies, as the softest pillows, the ones that give most, are frequently filled with down or other types of feathers. If you are allergic to these materials, you will develop a runny nose, sneezing and itchy eyes overnight, and, if you have asthma, you may cough or wheeze. This problem is particularly common in children with allergies. So, select your pillows carefully so that you can avoid the problems they sometimes create.

their body position throughout the night. The most common position for us to sleep in is on the right side, with the knees and hips slightly bent, and the second most common is the same position on the left side. Lying flat on your back with your arms crossed in front of you is the next most common position, though it has been noted that sleeping on your back throughout the night is generally associated with a poorer sleep than sleeping on your side. Sleeping on your stomach with your head turned to one side or another is the least common sleeping position.

Many people find it difficult to change the positions in which they sleep; for example, many wives know that their husbands tend to snore when sleeping on their backs and spend much of the night repeatedly jabbing and elbowing the sleeping husband into another position. Special pillows (such as those designed for neck pain) often reduce snoring, but success has also been achieved in changing people's favourite sleeping positions by simply trying to effect the change over ten days or two weeks rather than over a single night. It works like this. Let's say you normally sleep on your back, but you're aware that your snoring in this position disturbs your bed partner. Simply begin elevating one corner of your pillow (with a folded towel, for example) and sleeping on your back for a few nights with your pillow on this slight angle. Several nights later, increase the angle, so the pillow is now much higher on one side than the other. Your natural tendency will be to turn towards the side rather than remaining flat on your back. Simply repeat this process, gradually increasing the amount you raise the edge of the pillow, and in ten days or so you will be sleeping on your side naturally and your body will have easily adapted to the change. You must, of course, maintain the shape of the pillow to keep your head from falling back to the former position.

It's Not How You Sleep but with Whom

Helen Rowland, an American journalist, said, 'Before marriage, a man will lie awake thinking about something you said; after marriage, he'll fall asleep before you finish saying it.'

Could it be that your disturbed sleep comes from your bed partner?

Many couples sleep better when they sleep together; they are used to each other, and enjoy the physical closeness and security. Photography done in sleep laboratories of bed partners' movements in sleep overnight shows a choreography, a joint use of space. When one turns, the other often turns the same way. In this manner, physical touching (and thus sleep disturbance) is minimized.

However, a common problem couples experience is that the shared bed is far too small. A double bed occupied by two adults allows each of them about the same amount of space as a baby in a crib has, and sometimes this is just not enough. If your partner wakes up every time you turn over, you may need a larger bed – or even two beds pushed together. Sometimes, simply changing the size of the shared bed allows both partners a better sleep. Several studies have produced disturbing findings – namely, that many couples enjoy better-quality sleep when separated into single beds. These couples literally sleep better apart: they have more

---

Night Bites

Some people awaken in the middle of the night and simply cannot go back to sleep without eating. Occasionally a medical condition is the cause, but much more commonly, it's simply a learned habit – and a bad one at that. Unfortunately, waking at night to eat disturbs your sleep in several ways – first, by conditioning you to awaken in anticipation of the meal, and second, by setting in motion the digestive processes that disturb the remaining sleep by making it lighter and more fragmentary. You're better off eating well during the day, having only a glass of water if you need it at night.

Mae West, the screen actress, once said, 'I don't mind going to bed on an empty stomach – as long as it's not mine.' She was a very poor sleeper from all reports.

---

deep sleep, less frequent awakenings, and a more refreshing rest. Separate beds are particularly of benefit if the sleeping schedules of the couple are in conflict. If you need to go to bed early, and awaken early, yet your partner is a night owl and likes to sleep till noon, each of you may suffer trying to adapt to the other's sleep needs.

Especially if your bed partner disturbs your sleep with snoring, repeated movements and restlessness, or physical contact during the night, you might very well be able to enjoy a much more restful sleep in a separate bed, even in single beds pushed close together.

Sleep and Food

Mark Twain said, 'Part of the secret of success in life is to eat what you like and let the food fight it out inside,' but his advice may keep you awake all night.

There is good scientific evidence that what you eat can certainly affect your sleep. For many years it has been known that diets deficient in essential nutrients make people drowsy and fatigued, and also prevent them from having adequate sleep. Anorexia nervosa and bulimia, both chronic nutritional deficiency disorders, lead to poor sleep. Your diet must have all the essential nutrients to allow you to sleep well.

When we sleep seven and a half or eight hours, we usually fast as well. Yet this prolonged period without food or drink does not usually leave us overcome by hunger the next morning. Clearly, our nutritional needs are different when we are asleep and when we are awake. For this reason, having a heavy meal before you go to sleep disturbs the normal pattern of relative rest your digestive system takes during sleep. Consuming a large amount of food before bedtime results in enzymes being secreted to aid digestion during the night, and this process will interfere with your sleep.

Similarly, any food that produces increased acid secretion in the stomach may cause symptoms such as heartburn or gas during sleep. Spices, onions, peppers and other acid-producing foods have been shown to hamper sleep, and warm milk, Ovaltine (made from milk and cereal), Horlicks (a malt drink) or any food that is high in tryptophan (such as milk), before retiring, help people to sleep better. A meal high in carbohydrates (such as pasta) is much more soporific than one high in protein.

Many people find it difficult to stay awake immediately after lunch, and especially if lunch has been heavy, if they haven't slept well the night before, if the postlunch activities are dull or boring or if they consumed alcohol with their noon meal. Contrary to popular belief, the reason for this tiredness after lunch is not the lunch itself; volunteers who were tested for sleepiness were drowsier in this afternoon period than at any other time of the day except in the middle of the night, even when they had had no regular meals at all, just snacks every two hours during the day. The tendency to snooze after lunch occurs primarily because midday is the trough of your sleep–wake cycle, but the added effect of a large meal combines with the trough to produce an overwhelming effect. Having a lighter lunch, avoiding alcohol, being well rested the night before and including some stimulation such as movement in your early-afternoon routine will help alleviate the postlunch dip.

Sleep and Exercise

The relationship between physical activity and sleep is complex, but understanding the connections between the two is important if you want to improve the quality of your sleep.

Deep sleep is necessary for physical restoration. During deep sleep, the secretion of growth hormone reaches its daily peak, and in adults this hormone is responsible for tissue repair and renewal. Resting quietly in bed, awake, one is not able to achieve the same restorative function. Even sleeping lightly (in twilight-zone sleep) for extended periods does not achieve the same recovery. Accordingly, you would expect increased amounts of deep sleep after exercise, and this certainly is true in many cases – for example, marathon runners have a substantial increase in deep sleep on the evening after their event. Mild exercise, such as housework, bowling or

---

The Sleep of Olympians

Ever wonder how Olympic athletes sleep before their event? A study of ninety Olympic athletes on the U.S. Olympic team was done before the 1984 games. On average, team members slept about eight hours a day and most napped an average of one and a half hours as well. Only 3 per cent complained of significant insomnia when they were in training, but more than 50 per cent of them had difficulty sleeping before their competition, particularly the night before. As well, more than 60 per cent of them complained of the effects of jet lag and the timing of their specific events at international meets. Scheduling events so that athletes compete when they are at the most alert stage of their circadian rhythm is crucial to their performance. Unfortunately, some of the athletes must travel across several time zones to compete internationally – a disadvantage since they may have to participate in events at times not well suited to their bodies' schedule. Some athletes have to compete at a time that corresponds to the middle of the night for them. Understanding the importance of adequate sleep, athletes try to arrive in the country days, and sometimes weeks, ahead to get used to the new time schedule.

Even football and cricket teams, and other teams who have to travel, time their arrival very carefully to minimize sleep loss. A sleepy athlete simply cannot achieve his or her potential.

---

other light physical exertion, does not seem to make any difference to the subsequent amount of deep sleep. It appears that there is some threshold amount of energy that must be expended before the benefits of exercise are seen. These benefits include allowing you to go to sleep more quickly, increasing the amount of deep sleep and reducing the number of awakenings throughout the night. Good exercise makes you sleep better, and good sleep allows you to recover.

The benefits of exercise are not seen, however, if exercise is taken at the wrong time in relation to sleep. Essentially, you must time your exercise well if you want it to help you to sleep. Moderate physical activity just before you try to go to sleep actually disturbs sleep by delaying the onset of sleep and increasing the number of awakenings throughout the night. Optimally, you must exercise no less than four hours before trying to sleep. The best time to exercise is during the day or early evening; your body temperature may well be the reason.

Our body temperatures are not constant throughout the day; we have a built-in thermostat and our temperature increases to a maximum in midafternoon and then lowers very slowly to its minimum level at about four a.m. For most people, this change in temperature is just slightly less than one centigrade degree, though the change in temperature is less in older people. We sleep better when our temperature is falling than when it is at its peak, or rising. Most good aerobic exercise will increase your core temperature by about one centigrade degree and, after recovery, the temperature slowly falls back to the usual for that time of day. It seems that exercise too close to bedtime means that the temperature is still elevated when you are trying to sleep, and that's why exercise four to six hours before bedtime is ideal. There is some individual variation, but the principle applies: exercise earlier in the day or evening is better than exercise just before sleep. This may explain why a hot bath helps you sleep: the same principle applies – an increase in body temperature with a slow fall. A hot bath is more conducive to sleep if it occurs not immediately before bedtime, but an hour or so before.

BUT I DON'T LIKE EXERCISE

Robert Hutchins, an American educator, wrote, 'Whenever I feel like exercise I lie down until the feeling passes.' Many people share his opinion, approaching exercise as if it were drudgery. The first rule of exercise is that you must change your attitude towards it.

Exercise should be fun; the word our children use for it is *play*, and that is accurate. Ideally, exercise should be something that you enjoy, something that you look forward to and something that makes little demand on you mentally. It should be a stress-releasing time, not a stress-producing one. It should be a time for shedding the cares and worries of the day, when the mind is free to wander; it should not be an ordeal. The rhythmic movement of your body, especially outdoors, is an essential evolutionary requirement; that's what we as a species have been doing for millions of years. It's primal, and a basic human need. It's also fun.

What's the best exercise for you? The answer is: many different activities. Don't set yourself up with a programme of one single activity, such as jogging; no matter how much you think you enjoy it, if you do it frequently enough it will become tedious. Instead, develop an exercise schedule that involves doing many different activities. There is nothing more pleasing than mastering a new physical skill, such as rowing or playing tennis or bowls, no matter what your age. Explore those activities that you think you might like; you'll be surprised at the pleasure that accompanies learning a new sport.

Ideal exercise is aerobic – that is, sustained and uninterrupted – and lasts for at least twenty minutes a day. Such activities as brisk walking, bicycling, jogging, aerobic exercise routines, skiing, swimming and dancing qualify. Simple housework, garden work or similar activities usually do not produce the sustained effort that qualifies as adequate exercise and improves your sleep pattern. If you look at your daily activity schedule with a view to increasing the amount of time you devote to exercise, you'll find that the twenty minutes a day is easily accommodated. Soon you'll discover that exercise is not a chore, but an enjoyable part of your life.

5
Things That Go Bump in the Night

Sleepwalking

Sleepwalking is a spectacular and frightening event to witness. The blank expression, the seemingly purposeful movements, the automatic behaviour, the overwhelming sense that the person is not in touch with reality – all lend an eerie, out-of-this-world aura to the occurrence. Often, it is your loved ones that you observe in this mysterious state, which makes the event all the more disturbing. It's no wonder that sleepwalkers were once felt to be possessed, driven by a force, a spirit, other than their own. That this 'possession' occurs in the shadows of night and leaves no memory in the mind of the sleeper the next morning makes it even more puzzling, and somehow sinister.

A Sleepwalker's Nightmare

Michael, a thirty-seven-year-old car mechanic, had always

been strong and healthy, and had enjoyed heavy physical activity most of his life. He excelled at football, and had lately taken up long-distance running. He also enjoyed playing hard, and would often drink heavily. Everything in his life he approached with the same vigour and enthusiasm.

Michael came to my office to have stitches removed from his forearm. He wasn't his usual jovial self; he was a little sheepish, and was accompanied by his wife, Janet, who seemed clearly worried. He had a large ragged laceration on the front part of his forearm. As I took out the twenty-odd sutures, I asked him what had happened.

'Well, I'm not really sure,' said Michael. 'You'll have to ask my wife.' This was surprising, coming from a man who prided himself on being independent and self-sufficient.

Janet told me the story.

After a night of heavy drinking, in celebration of completing his latest marathon, Michael and his wife had fallen asleep in an inebriated state. The race had been held out of town, and they were staying at a hotel. About an hour after falling asleep, Janet was awakened by a noise. She was quite alarmed to see that Michael was out of bed and trying to open the sliding glass door to the small balcony of their fifth-floor room. She knew he had often sleepwalked in the past, but the episodes had usually consisted of his simply shuffling around in their bedroom with a kind of vague and purposeless movement, as if looking for something. She had always been able to talk him into quickly and cooperatively returning to bed.

This time was different. Janet was clearly upset as she recounted the story.

'Michael wasn't the same person. He was quite angry and, though I couldn't make out the exact words, it was clear he wanted out through that glass door. It was horrible!'

She tried to speak to him, then tried to lead him away from the door, but that seemed to upset him even more. He fumbled with the latch on the sliding glass door and, when he could not open it, frantically began searching the room. He grabbed a lamp that sat beside their bed and hit the door with it, breaking the glass. Cold air rushed in, and then she saw the blood. Michael was strangely silent and immobile, looking at his arm and then at the glass on the carpet. He seemed confused, disoriented.

'I began to cry, and then Michael seemed to snap out of it, telling me it was okay. He seemed himself again in a minute or two.' Janet was weeping as she relived the experience while describing it for me.

They stopped the bleeding by wrapping the cut forearm in a towel, then went to a hospital casualty department for stitches. Michael was unable to recall shattering the sliding glass door or having had any sort of dream.

The Nature of Somnambulism

The medical term for sleepwalking is 'somnambulism', derived from the Latin *somnus* (sleep) and *ambulo* (walk about). The phenomenon is not rare – in fact, it's almost universal in children. Most of us have had at least one episode of this nocturnal wandering, and some 15 per cent of children have recurring episodes. Though they can occur at any age after the child learns to crawl, most sleepwalking begins between the ages of four and twelve, with a peak incidence at age ten. Though it is very common in childhood, it is not common in adult life; fewer than one in two hundred adults are sleepwalkers. Somnambulism seems to be developmental and related to the depth of deep sleep in children. When it persists into adult life, the chances of harm, and the underlying causes, as we shall see, are different.

In childhood, the typical sleepwalking episode begins with the youngster sitting up soundlessly in bed. The child may pick at blankets or the bedclothes, look vacantly around the bedroom, and then simply lie back down and return to sleep. More commonly, the child rises from bed and begins to wander slowly around the room. The walking itself is deliberate, with little haste. Though the child looks straight ahead and seems to be on some kind of autopilot, there is a sense of purpose in the activity, some goal for the journey. Particularly in familiar surroundings, the child is well able to navigate in the dark, and usually avoids hitting walls and other obstacles. Sometimes he or she may turn on the light, get dressed or use the toilet (not always in the appropriate manner), though more complex actions are rare.

Sleepwalking children don't seem to be in any distress, or in any great hurry. Though they often give the impression they are looking for something, they're usually not agitated, and do not cry out. If they do speak at all (they rarely do, unless spoken to), they articulate poorly and the words are often incomprehensible or out of sequence. Vision appears to be intact, and they are able to avoid structures in their path. However, the brain is easily confused and certainly doesn't have the judgement and insight of wakefulness. Accidents can and do occur, especially in strange environments. If you speak to a sleepwalking child, he or she will often respond (though not always appropriately), and you can lead the child back to sleep quite easily. A light touch is often helpful. There seems to be no memory of the events in the morning; if the sleepwalking child is awakened, simple confusion results. He or she doesn't know what led to the journey to the hall, or what he or she was looking for.

How are we to understand these ghost-like behaviours in sleep?

In the sleep laboratory, researchers noted that sleepwalking occurs during the end of a period of deep sleep, just as the sleeper is rising into the lighter twilight zone of transitional sleep. For this reason, sleepwalking is considered by many to be a disorder of arousal. Sleepwalking, and its cousins sleep talking and night terrors, are all lumped together as 'partial arousals'. You will recall that the normal night's sleep begins with a descent into the so-called twilight zone, then further descent into deep sleep IV – the latter segment lasting approximately forty to forty-five minutes. After this period of sleep, there is a rise in the level of consciousness towards awakening. It is at this time that sleepwalking occurs. In deep sleep, remember, the brain is not functioning well; it's confused and befuddled if awakened.

It seems that in sleepwalking, the body wakes up before the mind does; the muscles are able to function (in walking and moving and so on) before the brain is wide awake and able to process external stimuli properly. This is why it's called a 'partial' arousal. The brain is still on 'cruise control'. During sleepwalking the brain waves exhibit a mixture of patterns – not wide awake, but not in deep sleep either. In a way, the body is fully awake and the brain is still partially asleep.

Children who are habitual sleepwalkers are more prone to the behaviour at times of increased stress and anxiety when fatigued. The explanation is thought to be that all of these factors cause an increase in deep sleep – the restorative phase of sleep – and somnambulism occurs on exiting this stage of sleep. Obviously, an increase in segments of deep sleep leads to more frequent exits from it, and therefore to more incidents of sleepwalking.

The likelihood of a child's sleepwalking increases tenfold if his or her parents or siblings are habitual sleepwalkers. Though sleepwalking episodes can increase in frequency during periods of stress, children who sleepwalk are usually not psychologically abnormal in any way, or more emotional or less stable than children who do not sleepwalk. The vast majority of youngsters who walk in their sleep will not continue the behaviour into adult life.

ADULT SLEEPWALKERS

Though adult sleepwalking is basically the same behaviour, linked with the same mechanism of partial arousal, it is not always as benign and innocent. It is more often associated with physical harm, as in Michael's case, because not only are adults larger and stronger, but also adult somnambulism tends to be more aggressive and adventurous. In addition, though adult sleepwalking is not necessarily a sign of an abnormal psychological state, there is more of an association with abnormal psychology.

What is known is that any factor causing an increase in heavy sleep will increase the chances of a sleepwalking incident. Heavy alcohol intake, as in Michael's case, excessive physical exertion or extreme fatigue increases the need for deep sleep, the stage associated with sleepwalking. Adults who sleepwalk have usually developed their pattern of abnormal sleep after age ten, and it usually lasts for years. Some adults show aggressive behaviour or anger during their sleepwalking episodes (it is unusual for children to do so) and, if so, psychological problems are more common.

Most sleepwalkers do not harm others, but they run the risk of harming themselves. This risk is especially high if, as Michael was, they are in an unfamiliar environment. It's as if the sleepwalker has 'memorized' the layout of his or her usual bedroom and house and is able to navigate safely around within that memory. Unfortunately, sleepwalking episodes often occur when people are away from home and cannot rely on memory. They fall off balconies, down stairwells, over furniture, into swimming pools, etc.

TIPS TO HELP SLEEPWALKERS

1. Most sleepwalking episodes, particularly in children, are short-lived and innocent and need no specific treatment. All that is necessary is to protect the youngster from harm. One should be very careful to lock the doors leading outside, using a child-proof mechanism. Similarly, an alarm system that is triggered by the opening of the child's bedroom door can be useful. The child's bedroom must be looked at carefully for potentially injurious objects or features. Windows are a potential source of danger, both from breaking glass and as a means of exit for the child. The room should contain no sharp objects, or piles of material that may topple and cause suffocation, or furniture that can be pulled over.

2. Adult sleepwalkers are as susceptible as children to the hazards mentioned above.

3. Most adults who sleepwalk are aware of the situations in which they are liable to do so – situations in which the amount of deep sleep is increased, including fatigue, sleep deprivation, excessive use of alcohol or other sedative drugs, and increased stress of any kind. The danger is always greater when the sleepwalkers are out of their usual environment, not only because of the disorientation during sleepwalking, but also because changes in the environment are often associated with a change in sleep pattern.

4. We know that the chance of sleepwalking is increased in

certain situations, and efforts to prevent sleepwalking episodes have been devised on the basis of that knowledge. Because sleepwalking occurs on exiting deep sleep, any drug that suppresses the amount of this sleep will also suppress the sleepwalking. Benzodiazepines and some antidepressants, such as imipramine, have this effect and are often very useful for adult sleepwalkers in strange or dangerous sleeping situations. Preventing excessive fatigue in sleepwalkers (especially children) will prevent the subsequent increase in deep sleep and help to decrease the chance of having a sleepwalking episode. Because stress is often a factor, and because a significant percentage of adult sleepwalkers have psychological difficulties, psychological counselling is often very effective, particularly for adults. Hypnosis has also been used to advantage, for similar reasons.

5. Excessive alcohol can cause or aggravate a tendency to sleepwalk, as can some medications – beta blockers, lithium, amitriptyline and certain sedatives and sleeping pills.

TIPS FOR SLEEPING WITH A SLEEPWALKER

1. If you sleep with a sleepwalker, you must know how to handle the phenomenon. First, if the sleepwalker is a child, you must realize that occasional sleepwalking is quite normal and of no great concern. It does not imply any underlying psychological problem, stress or other maladaptive behaviour. Children simply have more deep sleep than adults do, so their chance of sleepwalking is greater. You don't need to do anything except speak quietly to the child and direct him to return to bed. You can touch him lightly and guide him back to bed, tuck him in and he will usually cooperate, going back to sleep within a

few seconds. A characteristic of sleepwalking is amnesia – the sleepwalker is not awake, so in the morning will not remember that anything has happened at all. You have to be awake to remember. Don't mention the sleepwalking episode to the child. Don't tease him or joke about it. Doing so only makes the child wonder what sort of behaviour is going on beyond his control when the lights go out.

2. If you sleep with an adult sleepwalker, you should recognize the situations in which the sleepwalking is liable to occur. Though adult sleepwalking can be dangerous, most is not – and often, by talking quietly, you can direct the sleepwalker back to bed. It is not necessary to wake her and, in fact, waking only produces confusion. If the sleepwalker is not interested in returning to bed, rather

---

A Plea for Automatism

In the early hours of May 24, 1987, Mr Parks, a 27-year-old electrician, rose from sleep, left his home, and drove his car a distance of 14 miles (23 km) to the home of his parents-in-law.

Once there, he entered their house while they were sleeping, and with a kitchen knife attacked them in their beds. He stabbed his mother-in-law to death and seriously injured his father-in-law. Immediately after the incident, he drove to the nearby police station, again in his own car, and, in an agitated manner, told the police, 'Oh my God, I've just killed two people with my own hands. I stabbed and beat them to death. It's all my fault!'

At his trial for murder, the electrician pleaded automatism, stating that at the time he was sleepwalking. He had always slept poorly and had had significant increases in stress in the weeks preceding the death. Experts testified that he was in fact sleepwalking and that somnambulism is not a disease of the mind (that is, not an insanity), but simply a disorder of sleep. They also ruled that a sleepwalker's ability to voluntarily control his behaviour is 'severely limited or not available'.

He was found to be not guilty of any crime, as the court felt he was not responsible for his actions in this trance-like state.

than force the issue, you're best to simply protect her from physical harm. Usually there is only one episode of sleepwalking per night and this episode lasts often less than ten minutes.

3. Obviously if sleepwalking in adults is a recurring phenomenon, medical consultation should be obtained to rule out significant psychological or physical disease that could be treated. See your doctor.

Night Terrors

Cynthia was a perfectly normal, happy child – at least during the day. Like most seven-year-olds, she was cheerful and bubbly with a natural inquisitiveness, and she greeted each day with enthusiasm and energy. Her parents were both grateful and amazed that Cynthia had brought such joy into their lives. But there was no joy in their home when Cynthia went to bed.

Every night after they had tucked in their precious daughter, her anxious parents waited to see if she would have another one of her attacks. They listlessly watched television, or talked quietly, waiting for the awful sound – the scream that heralded another episode. The pattern was always the same. An hour or so after she went to sleep, Cynthia would suddenly sit bolt upright in bed and cry out. Her terrified parents would rush up into the bedroom to find their daughter sitting up in bed, her face flushed bright red, contorted with fear and covered with sweat. As she screamed she would sometimes throw the covers off her bed and wave her arms wildly in the air or pick repetitively at an imaginary object. Occasionally, and this was the most distressing to her parents, she would suddenly fly out of bed and rush around the bedroom, trying to avoid some unseen danger, all the while crying out in horror.

Her parents tried to talk to her and lead her back to bed, but Cynthia couldn't hear them, and resisted their attempts to resettle her. She acted as if she were possessed.

In spite of their intensity, the episodes were usually over in just a few minutes. Cynthia would become less agitated, often very quickly, and would return to her bed. She would lie down, yawn, and then fall fast asleep again. Her parents, drained by the experience, were astounded at how rapidly she could return to a deep and peaceful sleep.

In the morning, Cynthia was herself again. She never recalled the episode of the night before, and wondered why her parents seemed so concerned about what went on when she was asleep.

THE ANATOMY OF TERROR

Cynthia's attacks were night terrors, a particularly dramatic form of partial awakening from deep sleep. The proper name for night terror is *pavor nocturnus* (from the Latin *pavor*, meaning fear, and *nocturnus*, of course related to the night-time).

Night terrors most commonly occur in children between the ages of five and seven; though they can occur at any age, they are rare in adults. Ninety-six per cent of people who have night terrors have a family history of similar episodes, or of sleepwalking. In children, the terrors are not associated with any psychological problems whatsoever. In contrast, in adults, sleep terrors are often, though not always, associated with significant psychological abnormalities such as phobias, obsessive-compulsive disorders, depression, excessive agitation or stress.

Night terrors occur early in the night, usually as the child is exiting from the first period of deep sleep, often within one hour of going to bed. Like sleepwalking, the terror occurs in a situation of partial awakening; the brain is neither completely asleep nor completely alert. The most characteristic feature is that the terror is associated with intense fear and panic that produces the extreme anxiety with arousal, the flushed face, rapid heart beat, elevated blood pressure and other changes of a severe emotional response. Because the brain is only partially awake, children with night terrors will not respond to questions or instructions – they are not processing the input properly. Similarly, because the brain is not working normally, memory is not laid down, and the child will not recall the episode in the morning. Though night terrors are disturbing to watch, they are often short-lived and the child returns to sleep without difficulty. The episodes occur more frequently in children than in adults because, just like sleepwalking, they occur during deep sleep and of course children have more deep sleep than adults do. Any factor that increases deep sleep (such as fatigue) can increase the frequency of night terrors.

Night Terrors vs. Nightmares

It is important to distinguish night terrors from nightmares. The word nightmare comes from the old Saxon word *mara*, meaning demon. Nightmares are true dreams – that is, they occur during rapid-eye-movement sleep, not during deep sleep. Thus they tend to occur later in the night, and usually do not produce much physical reaction – as opposed to the loud screaming, flushed face, and rapid heart rate and breathing of the night terror. Nightmares occur when the body is paralyzed in REM sleep – only some twitching is seen and garbled sounds are heard, not the piercing scream that begins a night terror. When a child wakes up after a nightmare, he or she is perfectly wide awake, and able to be reasoned with and talked to normally. Usually the dream can be remembered in detail even in a young child, if questioning is done soon after the child awakens. With night terror, the child is very difficult to awaken and rarely will remember specific details – only the feeling of being frightened.

Cynthia was not aware of her night terrors, but she was aware that something was going on during sleep over which she had no control. All that was needed was to educate the parents about the benign nature of this seemingly dangerous and explosive type of occurrence. We ensured that Cynthia's demand for deep sleep remained constant by avoiding sleep-overs, staying up late, and other sources of disturbance in her sleep pattern. The episodes decreased in amount and, though still present, cause much less distress to the parents. They do not mention the episodes to Cynthia, who has forgotten about them.

TIPS TO HELP WITH NIGHT TERRORS

1. The same precautions to avoid injury in the sleeper must be observed as with sleepwalking. The room must be safe and predictable. Though night terrors often do not cause the sleeper to leave the bed, it is possible for him or her to suddenly and violently leap out of bed and move around the room, and the possibility for injury exists.

2. Though extremely frightening and disturbing to watch, we realize that night terrors in children are not associated with any specific medical or psychological problem. During the episode, in addition to protecting the sleeper, you may speak slowly and softly and sometimes this will allow the sleeping child to return to normal sleep. Most often though, the child does not seem to respond to you and all that's left is for you to simply wait until the episode

is completed and help the child back into bed and to sleep. As the episode ends, the child's brain actually enters the twilight zone – so the child may awaken, and may be surprised to find you looking so worried. As with sleepwalking, it's important to reassure the child that all is well and that there is no cause for alarm.

3. Night terrors in adults are more often associated with significant psychological disease or even illness – psychological assessment and consultation with a physician are strongly advised. As with sleepwalking, a low-dose benzodiazepine or imipramine (an antidepressant) can decrease the frequency of the episodes.

Sleep Talking

Talking in your sleep or, at least, making some sort of attempt at vocalization is extremely common, especially in children. It can be quite amusing to hear the confused mumblings of your child, but it can also be frightening. Though sleep talking can occur during any of the stages of sleep and at any time of the night, it's more common in twilight-zone sleep, especially when rising in alertness from deep sleep. Sleep talking is often associated with some movement of the sleeper – adjusting the pillow or the covers, rolling over in bed, and so on – and is sometimes associated with true sleepwalking.

Fully 20 per cent of episodes of sleep talking occur during REM or dream sleep, when the muscles of speech are normally paralyzed. These sleep-talking speech attempts are correlated with what the sleeper sees in his or her dream; if you wake up a sleeper soon after speech begins in REM sleep, more often than not he or she will tell you the content of the dream, and it will be relevant to the 'speech' that has just been uttered.

Contrary to popular belief, sleep talking, when it consists of meaningful words or phrases, does not reveal the hidden secrets of our deepest mind, but is usually more pedestrian. Most sleep talking simply reflects the day's activities, with talk of food, school work or discussions or meetings we might have had.

In fact, most sleep 'talk' is not organized but consists of a word or two, or perhaps a phrase or two – a disjointed thought or sentence. It's actually rather rare to get three or four sentences in a row; much more common is a single word such as 'righto' or 'good'; next most common is a short phrase or part of a sentence, an interrupted thought – such as 'All right then', 'It's ever so important', or 'I said no'. Quite commonly, there is some emotion or effect associated with the sleep talking; it can be anger or fear, but equally it can be joy or sadness.

Sleep talking during deep sleep, rather than REM sleep, usually consists of only a word or two, and these are often garbled or unintelligible, reflecting the depth of sleep.

CAN WE CONVERSE WITH SLEEP TALKERS?

As we have seen, most sleep talkers who utter intelligible sentences or phrases are in twilight-zone sleep. It is possible, though uncommon, to be able to have conversations with such a sleeper, including intelligible responses to questions asked by someone in the room with the sleeper.

UNDERSTANDING SLEEP TALKING

Sleep talking is not associated with any kind of psychiatric or psychological illness or, indeed, any other kind of illness. It seems to be simply a sort of malfunction, a glitch, whereby the decreased muscle tone that is usually present in the various stages of sleep is not achieved so that the sleeper is able to communicate partially. Sleep talking is just one more piece of evidence that some kind of thinking process is going on the entire night of sleep; and if the muscles are somehow allowed to react to this, sleep talking results. Though it is possible to reveal information during sleep talking, it is very rare. Sleep talking is benign, usually inconsequential and almost universal.

Grinding Your Teeth at Night

Forcible grating or gnashing of the teeth while asleep is called 'bruxism' (from the Greek *brucho*, meaning 'to grind or wear away'); it is a very common sleep complaint, but usually the one who complains is not the sleeper, for he or she does not wake up during the grinding, but anyone within earshot: the harsh scraping or rasping sound of tooth against tooth is very loud and quite characteristic. Bruxism is caused by the repetitive contraction of the large jaw muscles, which forces the teeth to rub violently together, and it occurs in at least 15 per cent of the adult population and up to 25 per cent of children. Bruxism knows no age limits, occurring in children less than a year old, and in the elderly, who, after losing their teeth, are known to gnash their gums all night or even grind their dentures! Though the sleeper is not aware of the sound (it's an impressive noise, but oddly doesn't wake up the one who's making it), he or she often experiences an aching pain in the jaw area – characteristically in the area where the jaw joins the skull, just in front of the ear – or a headache, in the morning.

The force involved in repeated nocturnal teeth grinding

can be quite severe. Inflammation of the gums, stretching of the temporomandibular joint of the jaw, arthritis in the jaw and even a thinning of the bone of the jaw have all been reported. Jaw-muscle and tooth sensitivity are common, but sometimes the pain is more difficult to localize. Many people simply complain of a sore ear or even a sore neck. Sometimes the dentist makes the diagnosis; the grinding literally wears down the teeth, rubbing off the enamel and loosening the support for the teeth in the bones of the jaw. The reported incidence of bruxism in dental patients is 20 per cent, and about 10 per cent of these patients need specific repair to their teeth to fix the abnormal wear or damage to the surrounding tissues.

Grinding of the teeth during the day is quite uncommon, although it is seen in some severe psychiatric illnesses, in brain damage of whatever cause and in mental retardation.

Nocturnal bruxism occurs in episodes throughout the night, and each episode is fairly short, lasting four to five seconds, but very violent. Episodes most commonly occur during light, or twilight-zone sleep, though overnight studies have recorded incidents during every sleep stage, including dream sleep.

The violent contractions of the jaw muscles during nocturnal tooth grinding produce the unmistakable sound. These contractions are not voluntary; during the day it is impossible voluntarily to contract your muscles with sufficient force to reproduce the sound in all its intensity. It is only during sleep that the full force of these muscle contractions is seen.

CHEWING ON YOUR PROBLEMS ALL NIGHT LONG

There is some debate about what causes nocturnal tooth grinding. There is certainly a tendency for the behaviour to run in families, which indicates some kind of genetic predisposition. Dentists report that specific anatomical or dental factors in the jaw often predispose a patient to bruxism – for example, malocclusion (where the teeth of the upper jaw do not fit well with the teeth of the lower jaw). In addition, alcohol consumption can lead to bruxism, actually causing it to occur in people who do not normally grind their teeth.

However, there is universal agreement that episodes of bruxism increase with stress. Studying for a final examination, a deterioration in an interpersonal relationship, a new job, and many other stressful situations have been shown to increase the frequency of episodes of nocturnal teeth gnashing, or even to produce them in people not normally given to bruxism. There is no doubt about it – we chew over our problems at night.

Though stress can increase bruxism, psychological profiles of those who grind their teeth are no different from those of the general population. Tooth grinders tend to obsessional personality features and to both anxiety and anger, especially suppressed or unexpressed anger, but they are usually not psychologically ill; they are often high achievers.

The causes of bruxism are not clearly defined, but what is known is that the tendency to grind your teeth at night is a fairly innocent behaviour, except for the damage that it does to your teeth. We also know that it gets worse with increased stress, but it is not a reflection of a significant underlying disease.

TIPS FOR TEETH GRINDERS
1. See your dentist. He or she will assess whether or not there is a dental or anatomical cause for your tooth grinding and correct it. Also, he or she will assess the damage to your teeth, as well as the periodontal tissues

that support the teeth. The most common accepted treatment for bruxism is some sort of tooth guard to protect them at night – a plastic or rubber pad that is moulded to the shape of your teeth. The guard doesn't stop the grinding motions, but does stop the damage to the teeth.

2. Try to decrease your stress. Do you have some suppressed anger? If so, you may be able to reduce your teeth grinding by identifying the source of your frustration and making some attempt to deal with it.

3. Restrict your consumption of alcohol, because it aggravates bruxism, or even causes it.

4. Teeth grinding may very well be the cause of that regular early-morning headache (especially in the temples), or the ache in your jaw or ears on arising. Ask family members if they have heard the characteristic sound of grinding teeth or have been diagnosed themselves. Then consult with your doctor to treat these secondary symptoms of tooth grinding.

5. Sometimes bruxism is caused or aggravated by medications such as sleeping pills or antidepressants.

6
Narcolepsy: Seizures of Sleep

As soon as she regained consciousness after the accident, Julia's first concern was not for herself, but for her children. The car had come to rest on its roof, and Julia was hanging upside down, her seat belt still fastened. She could hear crying coming from the back of the vehicle, and she quickly untangled herself. Crawling along the roof of the car, she found her daughter, Sarah, age two, still strapped securely in her car seat and unhurt. Andrew, age five, had already undone his belt and was softly whimpering, frightened but not injured. Julia got them both outside the ruined car before the enormity of it all hit her. Sobbing, she held her children tightly in her lap until the ambulance arrived.

I first met Julia a few minutes later in the casualty department, when, still shaken, she told me the story. 'I guess I must have fallen asleep . . . again' was how she put it.

There had been no other vehicle involved, and the road was clear and dry. It was midafternoon on an early spring day. Julia had not been drinking, and the motorway had been deserted. In fact, these conditions probably contributed to the accident because they let Julia begin to relax her guard while driving, to allow her mind to wander and to decrease her awareness of the external environment, in short, to begin to fall asleep. She had simply let the car drift towards the side of the road; when the tyres caught on the soft gravel, Julia suddenly awoke, jerked the steering wheel over to regain the pavement, and the vehicle flipped over and rolled several times.

Even a momentary lapse of attention, just the very beginning of twilight-zone sleep, can have disastrous consequences. The cost in terms of lost lives, human suffering and damages is staggering. The Department of Transport estimates that 20 per cent of all major car crashes are due to the driver falling asleep. These crashes tend to be more serious as no evasive action is taken.

Julia had fallen asleep other times as well – many other times. She seemed to be tired all day long and would fall asleep predictably when watching television or when trying to read a book after supper. She would fall asleep quite regularly in cinemas, in meetings or after a heavy meal, especially lunch. She was aware that she tended to fall asleep whenever she was in a quiet setting, no matter what time of day. On several occasions she had caught herself dozing off while driving – not actually falling asleep but on the way to it – and she would stop the car, open the window for some fresh air or get out and go for a short walk.

Sometimes though, she was simply unable to prevent sleep, even in an inappropriate setting. She just couldn't seem to help herself. Once she had embarrassed herself terribly by falling asleep while playing cards with friends – her head had fallen forward onto the card table!

In the casualty department, she told me about her other symptoms – her 'spells'. She described frightening episodes of total body weakness, like a paralysis, that came without warning. She would feel as if all her muscles had relaxed – had given way – and her head would fall forward, her arms and hands would go loose and her legs would buckle. She would, of course, drop whatever she was holding in her hands, and often she would fall to the floor, though sometimes, during minor spells, she would be able to catch herself as she was falling, and her muscles seemed to regain control. She was always wide awake during the spells, never dizzy or light-headed, and she never knew when or where they would occur. She found them terrifying, and they seemed to be increasing in frequency. On one occasion, Julia was scolding the family dog for tracking dirt into the kitchen, then suddenly found herself falling and, unable to catch herself, landed flat on the floor beside the bewildered poodle. She was unable to move for only a few seconds, but it seemed like an eternity.

Only after specific questioning did she admit to another problem – that, on occasion, she would awake from sleep and be unable to move, though her mind was active and alert. She knew she was awake; she could hear and feel, but she could not move a muscle, open up her eyes or speak. She wondered if these episodes meant that she was developing some form of mental illness.

Julia was found to have a sleep disorder called 'narcolepsy', which was the cause of her accident and the other symptoms. The disease allows us, through its manifestations, to understand better the nature of human sleep; it is an example of what happens when the complex process of sleep becomes disrupted.

Seizures of Sleep

The word 'narcolepsy' is derived from two Greek words:

narkosis, meaning a benumbing, or sleep; and *lepsis*, meaning a sudden occurrence, a seizure. The medical term 'narcolepsy' was coined by a French physician named Gélineau, who, in 1880, first described recurring episodes of unavoidable sleep – literally, of 'sleep attacks'. These episodes, Gélineau observed, came on as suddenly and as unpredictably as epileptic seizures, or convulsions. The patient would fall to the ground without warning, as would someone experiencing an epileptic seizure, but instead of the shaking of the limbs characteristic of epileptic seizure, sleep attacks involved no movement, just sleep. We now know that narcolepsy has nothing to do with epilepsy or true seizures, but is a disorder of sleep.

Before the First World War, narcolepsy was considered to be quite rare, but the encephalitis epidemics of 1917–1922 produced many cases and, as a result, the understanding of the disease grew. It was learned that there are four classical symptoms: excessive daytime sleepiness with attacks of irresistible sleep, drop attacks (or cataplexy), sleep paralysis and sleep-related hallucinations. Many patients with narcolepsy do not have all these symptoms, but nearly all narcoleptics have excessive daytime sleepiness – the tendency to fall asleep quickly when the environment is quiet or nonstimulating.

Narcolepsy is fairly common, occurring about as frequently as multiple sclerosis – that is, one case in a thousand people. It is as common in men as in women and, though the exact cause is not known, there is a genetic predisposition; both narcolepsy and excessive sleepiness are more common in relatives of patients with narcolepsy than in the general population. However, it is not simply an inherited disease. Though it can be caused by viral infections (such as those responsible for the encephalitis epidemics in 1917–22), head injuries, and (rarely) brain tumours, most narcolepsy is now felt to be due to an autoimmune disease process. The disease commonly begins in adolescents and young adults, and the first symptom is usually excessive sleepiness. Like Julia, these young people fall asleep easily at any time during the day, which may be their only symptom until many years later. Curiously, in at least half of the cases, the symptoms begin after some disruption to sleep pattern, such as a change in the sleep–wake cycle, a traumatic emotional event (such as the death of a spouse or other tragedy) or some other stress that affects sleep.

All patients with narcolepsy have excessive daytime somnolence, and most develop sleep attacks over the course of many years. Many narcoleptics develop drop attacks, sleep paralysis, and sleep-related hallucinations, though these symptoms may not all be present in every case.

The symptoms of narcolepsy are so insidious that the disorder has the dubious distinction in medical circles of being the disease that takes the longest time interval between initial presentation and diagnosis. In one series it took an incredible ten years from the time patients first began to experience problems until the correct medical diagnosis was made.

An Understanding of Narcolepsy

Though the full mechanism of the disease of narcolepsy is not understood, an abnormality of REM sleep, the sleep of dreams, is thought to be the problem. Simply put, in narcolepsy inappropriate REM sleep intrudes into wakefulness, creating a desire for REM sleep so powerful that it cannot be denied. Remember, REM sleep is associated not only with vivid dreams, but also with paralysis of most of the major muscle groups of the body. This understanding of the inappropriate intrusion of REM sleep into wakefulness explains many of the clinical manifestations of the disease. It seems as though the brain of a patient with narcolepsy harbours an intense desire for REM sleep, lurking just beneath the surface and waiting for any opportunity to capture the function of the brain.

In the sleep laboratory, patients with narcolepsy fall asleep very quickly, but instead of entering deep sleep the way normal subjects would, quickly enter REM sleep – often within only a few minutes. (Remember, normally the first REM sleep episode of the night occurs about ninety minutes after retiring.) It's as if narcoleptics must have REM sleep immediately. Over the course of the night, their amount of deep sleep is very much reduced (that's why they're chronically sleep deprived), their number of wakenings is greatly increased, but the total amount of REM sleep is normal.

During the day, individuals with narcolepsy have an excessive drive to sleep. In addition, people with narcolepsy have episodes when the REM sleep lying just beneath the surface of their alert state actually intrudes into wakefulness – pushes its way into control of the brain and forces them into the dream-like state of REM sleep. This explains the sleep attack Julia had when she was driving. She wasn't driving, she was dreaming – in REM sleep that would not be denied.

The drop attacks and sleep paralysis are thought to be related to an abnormality in REM sleep as well. Both these symptoms represent partial episodes of REM sleep, involving only the paralysis part of the sleep, not the dreams. It's as if the overpowering urge for REM sleep that is characteristic of narcoleptics has only partially taken over the brain and has achieved the paralysis of REM sleep without the sleep itself.

Many patients with narcolepsy are excessively sleepy most

of the time. They could easily drift off at the cinemas, watching television, attending an after-dinner lecture or in any other situation where the stimulation is minimal and sleep is, though not socially acceptable, not entirely inappropriate.

However, when Julia fell asleep at the card game with her face resting on the table, this was clearly inappropriate sleep. Several times a day, narcoleptics endure the sudden onset of these irresistible urges. These attacks can occur anytime – while eating, working, driving – and often during activities that normally would preclude sleep. Though the sleep may last as long as an hour if the subject is in a comfortable position, the sleep attack usually lasts a much shorter time, only a few minutes perhaps, and the patient wakes up refreshed. There seems to be a refractory period after such a sleep, lasting one to two hours, during which time the narcoleptic will not have another sleep attack. With EEG monitoring, brain activity during these sleep attacks has been found to be characteristic of REM-type sleep.

Cataplexy: Drop Attacks

Julia's description of the episode of falling on her kitchen floor when scolding her poodle was typical of cataplexy, or drop attacks, another symptom of narcolepsy. The word 'cataplexy' comes from the Greek *kata*, meaning down, and *lepsis*, meaning seizure, and is a symptom manifested by 70 to 90 per cent of people with narcolepsy.

Basically, drop attacks are sudden, unavoidable episodes of muscle paralysis, causing loss of postural tone. They are thought to be the result of REM sleep intruding on wakefulness, except they involve no sleep, just the paralysis that usually accompanies REM sleep. During these attacks, narcoleptics are fully awake and conscious, but feel their muscles loosen and give way suddenly. Sometimes this produces just the fleeting sensation of weakness, or perhaps a momentary partial loss of tone in one muscle group – a drooping of the head, a brief stutter, a buckling of the knees or a weakening of the grasp of a hand. Sometimes, however, as in Julia's kitchen, it produces a total powerlessness and collapse, a fall to the ground, perhaps leading to injury. The episodes rarely arise on their own, but the precipitating factor is often a strong emotional reaction such as anger or excitement. Even pleasant emotions such as joy or elation can cause the response; curiously, laughter is one of the commonest triggers. Because most cataplectic episodes are mild and short, they may appear to the observer (or even to the patient) to be only momentary lapses – perhaps categorized as clumsiness or being accident-prone.

Sleep Paralysis: The Living Zombie

Up to 50 per cent of narcoleptics experience paralysis associated with sleep. The episodes occur just at sleep onset or on awakening. In either case, the subject is awake, and aware, but cannot move – can't talk, roll over, lift a hand, call out, even open up the eyelids to see. These episodes of total paralysis are short, lasting only one to four minutes, but are often associated with the last of the classic symptoms of narcolepsy – vivid hallucinations – that make the episodes of paralysis even more terrifying. Though they can be simple benign images, the hallucinations of narcolepsy are often wild and bizarre, nightmare-like events and, when they occur with sleep paralysis, usually produce extreme anxiety. Many patients find themselves bombarded with brightly coloured images, loud noises and frightening experiences – for example, the feeling of moving in space or floating above the bed – combined with a total inability to move.

In African and Caribbean cultures, the word 'zombie' is used to describe a corpse brought back to life by magical powers, and these narcoleptic hallucinations, when they occur with sleep paralysis, are among the most frightening of human experiences – with the horribly graphic bombardment of images, combined with the corpse-like inability to move or react at all. These 'dreams' are all the more terrifying, as the subject is not even asleep but wide awake, and aware of the surroundings and of the unreality of the images.

Sleep paralysis is not specific to narcolepsy; perfectly normal people can have occasional episodes of sleep paralysis, usually without hallucinations.

With the combination of horrible and bizarre hallucinations, sleep and drop attacks, and paralysis on awakening, no wonder many patients with narcolepsy fear that they are mentally ill.

Other Features of Narcolepsy

Headache is a very common symptom in narcolepsy, as is memory loss, lethargy and inability to concentrate, all resulting from chronic sleep deprivation. Automatic behaviour, the performance of routine tasks by a person who is not consciously controlling the activity, is also common. A period of increased drowsiness usually precedes the automatic behaviour, and it often occurs when a person is doing some repetitive, monotonous task. Though the person is able to complete the activity (often not completely correctly), he or she may actually have been asleep for part of the time and may not recall having done the activity when awakened afterwards. Automatic behaviour is not specific to narcolepsy, but it reinforces the narcoleptic's lack of self-trust and lack of dependability.

Depression is a common consequence of the illness, as narcolepsy obviously interferes with one's ability to perform many normal human activities, such as holding a steady job, driving a car, operating machinery, attending meetings and looking after young children. Many of these patients are considered to be slothful and lacking in interest or self-motivation. It is to be emphasized that narcolepsy is a disease and beyond the patient's control, and is a lifelong affliction.

Tips for Narcoleptics

Narcolepsy is not simply a variant of normal sleep but, rather, a significant sleep disorder, literally a disease of sleep, and it is impossible to diagnose without a consultation with a physician and a sleep study. If you suspect you may have narcolepsy, see your doctor. Though no specific cure for narcolepsy is known, the disorder can be managed with a physician's assistance.

1. Maximize the efficiency of your sleep. You need a regular sleep schedule, going to sleep and awakening at specific times – to protect your deep sleep and prevent excessive daytime sleepiness. Avoid shift work, irregular schedules, late nights and variable wake-up times.
2. Use short daytime naps to your advantage. Because narcoleptics are usually at their most alert after a nap, schedule short rests before important meetings or activities. In many cases, a regular nap two or three times a

day will improve efficiency and prevent sleep attacks. Such naps need not be long (fifteen to twenty minutes is often enough) and can be accommodated by most work schedules.

3. Increase physical activity and avoid boring or repetitive tasks during those times when you are least alert (such as the afternoon circadian sleep–wake trough between 2:00 and 4:00 p.m.). The tendency towards sleep attacks is enhanced by high temperatures, indoor activity, idleness, heavy meals and boring or repetitive tasks in a nonstimulating environment. These factors should be avoided, but if that is impossible, they should be scheduled for your most alert periods of the day.

4. Avoid alcohol and other sedatives (such as antihistamines) as they aggravate many of the symptoms of narcolepsy.

5. Use caffeine to increase your alertness, bearing in mind that caffeine use may interfere with your obtaining deep sleep (particularly if the caffeine intake occurs in the later part of the day), though it can help keep you awake earlier.

6. Avoid dangerous activities such as swimming, cooking, driving, and handling machinery. People with narcolepsy should be aware of the importance of particular vigilance when looking after infants. No matter how hard you try, you may not be able to protect yourself or others from the onset of irresistible sleepiness, or a loss of muscle control or coordination that could be disastrous. Because cataplexy and sleep attacks are unpredictable, caution must be exercised at all times.

7. If you and your doctor decide to use medicines to treat narcolepsy, some sort of stimulant is the mainstay of treatment. Drugs such as modafinil, dexamphetamine and mazindol are examples of stimulating medicines used to

decrease the frequency of sleep attacks and excessive day-time drowsiness. Drugs such as clomipramine, an antidepressant, can be used to treat the drop attacks of cataplexy, as well as sleep paralysis and hallucinations. Sometimes sleeping pills, especially short-acting ones, are used to improve the quality of nighttime sleep.

8. The psychological consequences of narcolepsy may be significant but are avoidable. It is important to try to avoid feelings of guilt, inadequacy, anger and depression. Try to address this component of the illness by learning all you can about narcolepsy – no one has as much to gain from a thorough understanding of the disease as you. Self-help groups are excellent sources of information and support (see Further Resources).

Tips for Those Who Live with a Narcoleptic

1. If you suspect that your partner has narcolepsy, convince him or her to see his/her doctor. A diagnosis of narcolepsy is not lightly made and may require an objective evaluation of sleep pattern.

2. Understand that narcolepsy is a true sleep disorder, an actual disease involving sleep. The signs and symptoms are not within the voluntary control of those who have the disease; they are not lazy, uninterested, shifty, untrustworthy or manipulative, any more than any other person. They need your support and understanding.

3. Educate family, friends and employers about the disease, its special needs (such as daytime naps), and its physical (not psychological) basis. Simple adjustments in schedules and responsibilities can allow people with narcolepsy to participate normally in life.

4. Try to make changes in daily routines to protect nightly sleep (for example, by keeping regular sleeping hours), as

well as allowing nap times during the day and before events requiring complete alertness.

5. The sleep paralysis of narcolepsy can often be reversed quickly simply by touching the person who is paralyzed.

6. To protect people with narcolepsy from injury, you will have to share the responsibilities for driving, operating machinery and caring for children.

7. Though there is no specific cure for narcolepsy, understanding the mechanisms of the disease, making adjustments to the daily routine, protecting the nighttime sleep, and using medication all enable narcoleptics and their families to have much happier and fulfilling lives.

7
Movement Disorders in Sleep

In her dream, Agnes was no longer the aging widow she was in real life, but a young girl again, in the big old house where she had grown up so happily. She dreamed she was standing with her back to the living-room fireplace, warming herself in the cheerful heat of the blaze that crackled behind her. She could feel the tingle on the back of her legs, as if the fire itself were dancing lightly on her skin. The feeling of her childhood, a warm and happy calm, spread over her.

Suddenly, in the dream, the heat of the fire was no longer pleasant. Something was wrong. She could feel a burning pain, beginning in her leg. She tried to pull away, but couldn't. Her leg was paralyzed, and the terrible pain increased, scorching into her dream. She couldn't move, though the burning became worse and worse.

As she awoke, Agnes realized that the throbbing pain in her leg was not a dream at all, but simply another excruciating cramp in the muscles of her calf, just like the ones she had had on many, many previous nights. Struggling out of bed, she tried to stand, but the muscles were rigidly in spasm, and she moved only with great pain. She tried to massage the knotted mass in her lower leg to begin to release the agonizing contraction, and she could feel the tender hardness of the area. After a while, she was able to stand on the cold bedroom floor and stretch out the angry muscles. It was 2:30 a.m., and Agnes faced another sleepless night.

All her life Agnes had had more energy than the people around her. She simply felt better if she was very active and, even in retirement, she filled her days with many different activities. When her husband had died, she felt that being busy would help her to keep going. He had often said of her that she just couldn't sit still, and Agnes knew that this was quite true – she found it very difficult simply to sit quietly with nothing to do. Even as a young adult, Agnes hadn't been able to sit still for long: her legs became too uncomfortable, with an awful feeling inside them that disappeared as soon as she moved them, bounced them up and down or got up and walked. She derived no peace, no calm, from sitting quietly during the day, so she rarely did.

But lately, her nights were becoming unbearable. Far too frequently, her sleep was broken violently by the cramping in her legs or feet, and even if she didn't actually awake with the dreadful tightening in the muscles, she seemed to be a restless sleeper. In the morning the bed looked like she had spent the entire night twisting and turning; even the mattress cover pulled loose. When Agnes finally came to my office asking for help with her sleep, she wanted me to stop all the activity she had at night, the tossing and turning, so she would be able to once again arise each morning refreshed, rested enough to allow her to participate fully in her active life. She wanted the energy she wasted at night made available to her during the day.

Rocking and Rolling the Whole Night Through

Some degree of movement is an essential part of a normal night's sleep. Such actions as rolling from side to side, stretching out and then flexing up your arms and legs, and adjusting the covers and pillow are all natural and necessary. These types of movement occur on average about once every fifteen to twenty minutes during sleep, usually at the end of a period of deep sleep or REM sleep, when sleep is shallower and we enter twilight-zone or light sleep. Most of these movements are not sufficient to cause awakening, so we're not aware of them in the morning, even though they occur all night long. These turnings and shiftings prevent skin breakdown from prolonged local pressure. They also help to maintain body temperature (by adjusting the coverings over the body and the positioning of the limbs), and protect us from the consequences of prolonged immobility. Such problems as damage to superficial nerves from direct pressure, local congestion caused by poor circulation due to the obstructed drainage of blood, and overnight damage to tendons and ligaments from prolonged overstretching are all eliminated by this simple remedy – regular changing of position while still asleep.

We use the phrase 'sleep like a log' to describe a perfect sleep, one that is deep and undisturbed, but, in fact, to sleep like a log – totally immobile and unresponsive to the environment – could be disastrous. Imagine that you fell asleep on your side, with your arm and hand lying directly under your chest, and suppose you slept 'like a log' for seven and a half hours, and literally did not move at all during the entire time.

When you awoke, your arm and hand would be very sore

from having been immobile all night and from the cramped positioning. You would have pumped arterial blood into the arm and hand all night, but the weight of your chest pressing down on it would have impaired the drainage of venous blood out of the limb, so your hand, and especially your fingers, would be quite swollen. The pressure on your skin where it touched the mattress would have been enough to blanch out the blood supply to these areas, so you would have several large ugly bruised areas on the skin – perhaps even ulceration with loss of skin where it touched the mattress. The nerves in your arm might be damaged as well, and you might awaken unable to move your hand, or with a peculiar tingling or numbness in the hand caused by local pressure (from the weight of your body) on the nerves that course to the skin's surface, unprotected by muscles or other padding.

Some movement, some turning and shifting throughout the night, is a necessary and protective component of sleep.

Numbness in the Night: Pressure Palsies

Have you ever woken up with numbness or tingling in your arms or hands? This disconcerting symptom leads many to fear that they're having a stroke or heart attack, or suffering some other medical calamity. The usual story is that you are enjoying a nice deep slumber, when your sleep is interrupted by a strange and disturbing feeling in your hands or arms. It is usually described as a tingling or a numbness, but sometimes it can feel like a weak electrical shock or even a pulsing throb. When you awaken and try to move the arm or hand, you can't move it normally and it feels numb when you touch it with your other hand. Your concern wakes you up fully, and you shake the arm and hand and try to get it moving. Over the next couple of minutes, warmth and feeling return to the hand quite quickly, though not always completely, and you're able to return to sleep again. Sometimes the episodes will recur repeatedly in a single night.

As disturbing as these episodes are, they're innocent; they're palsies caused simply by pressure on superficial nerves. When you're asleep, the posture that you have adopted has put pressure on one of the superficial nerves to your arm or hand. This local pressure on a superficial nerve has interrupted the flow of impulses along the course of the nerve, and the nerve complains, sending sensations of altered feeling (the numbness and tingling) down the course of the nerve into your arm or hand. When you awaken and change position the pressure is relieved and, fairly quickly, the function of the nerve returns and feeling comes back. There are three common variants:

1. *The Funny Bone.* The ulnar nerve (*ulna* is Latin for 'forearm') comes to just beneath the surface of the skin on the inside of your elbow. You can easily feel it yourself by pressing behind the bony prominence on the inside of the elbow. This is called the 'funny bone' because, when you press on the nerve, it sends a 'funny' electrical-type shock into the hand. If you sleep on your back, for example, with your arms at your sides, the elbow will lie unprotected on the mattress. This can produce local pressure on the ulnar nerve at the elbow and produce a characteristic ulnar palsy – probably the most common numbness or tingling that awakens sleepers. The numbness, tingling and electrical feeling occur over the little finger and one-half of the ring finger (the half away from the thumb), the path of the ulnar nerve in the hand, and these two fingers won't work well.

2. *Saturday-Night Palsy*. The radial nerve lies on the inside of the arm and is quite close to the skin halfway between the shoulder and the elbow. It, too, is liable to be affected by pressure. Pressure on this area produces numbness on the back of the wrist and, more disturbingly, an inability to extend or lift up the wrist or to straighten the fingers out. This injury to the radial nerve has been called 'Saturday-night palsy' because it has been observed in inebriated revellers who spend the night asleep with their arm over the back of a chair.

3. *Carpal Tunnel Syndrome*. At the level of the wrist (in Latin, *carpos*), there is a tight anatomical space, or 'tunnel', made up of the bones of the wrist on the roof and a tight gristle on the floor. Through this 'tunnel' passes the median nerve of the forearm, as well as many of the tendons that make the fingers work.

Any increase in pressure within this 'tunnel' puts pressure on the nerve, causing dysfunction within the nerve and subsequent tingling and numbness downstream. It is a very common cause of discomfort in the hands at night. The sensation is typically described as severe numbness over the palm, the thumb, and the index and middle fingers, but it is often accompanied by some pain in the region of the wrist and even up into the forearm. Carpal tunnel syndrome often occurs in people who use their hands a lot – carpenters and mechanics and computer operators, though it is quite common among pregnant women and also in those whose thyroid function is less than normal. The numbness and tingling seem to be much worse at night, probably because of the position the wrists are in when you sleep. Many people sleep with their arms close to their chest and their elbows and wrists flexed, and this increases the pressure within the carpal tunnel, causing the sensation. Sometimes carpal tunnel syndrome cannot be relieved simply by movement at night, and medical treatment or surgery is required to correct it completely.

4. *Other Causes of Numbness and Tingling.* Stretching of any superficial nerve or local pressure on exposed nerves can cause almost any number of other episodes of numbness and tingling. Neck disease often causes pressure on the nerves that go to the arms, particularly in REM sleep, when the neck muscles are most relaxed. Similarly, many people with sciatica (pain along the sciatic nerve leading from the lumbar, or lower back, area) find that they waken with aggravated symptoms during the night if their sleeping position stretches the nerve.

Many people sleep with their arms in an unusual or uncomfortable position, such as flexed under their head or even over their head. Such positions often put a stretching-type pressure on the nerves of the shoulder and the arm radiating from the neck area. All of these common palsies can be prevented by paying careful attention to sleeping posture, and to the surface on which you sleep.

Nocturnal Leg Cramps

When Agnes awoke from her dream of childhood, the severe pain that she felt in the back of her leg was a nocturnal muscle cramp. A cramp is simply a painful, prolonged and unwanted contraction of muscle.

Cramping in the legs at night is one of the most common causes of disturbed sleep, especially among older people. In one study of those over fifty years of age, more than 70 per cent experienced leg cramps at least once a week. It is not a disease, but recurring leg cramps cause much unnecessary suffering, from both the pain and the disruption of sleep.

Most muscle tightenings don't hurt; the pain in a cramp is caused by several factors. First, the muscle shortens so violently that waste products are generated within the muscle and produce pain. Second, the muscle is working so hard that the body is unable to provide it with an adequate blood supply; the muscle being relatively starved of blood is another source of pain. Finally, in severe cramp, the muscle itself may be damaged, with partial tearing of microscopic parts of the individual muscle fibres.

A muscle lives a fairly simple life. It can do only two things: shorten (that is, contract) or lengthen (that is, relax). Shortening is an active process, usually occurring when the muscle gets the appropriate signal from a nerve. Lengthening is passive and, normally, muscles function in opposing pairs – for the muscles of one side of a joint to contract, the muscles on the other side of the joint must relax.

DO-IT-YOURSELF CRAMP

When we apply this idea of muscles working in opposing pairs to the ankle, we can see that the muscles at the back of the calf (the large amount of muscle tissue behind and below your knee), when shortened, cause the ankle to bend and the sole of the foot to move down, towards the floor. It's the action of going from standing flat on your feet to standing on your toes, and is the ankle motion necessary for walking. For this shortening to occur, the opposing muscles, those at either side and in front of the shin bone, must relax. These muscles are not as large as those at the back of your calf, because lifting the toes and the foot to take another step does not require as strong a muscle as pushing down against the ground and lifting the entire weight of the body while walking, which is what the large muscles of the calf do. Nevertheless, the muscles that cause your toes to lift up are opposing muscles to those that cause your toes to bend away from you.

In most joints, when a muscle on one side contracts, the muscle on the opposite side produces some drag as it lengthens, some force resisting the contraction of the other muscle. Remember, lengthening of muscle is a passive phenomenon, and in fact, the muscle on one side of the joint is lengthened by active shortening of the muscle on the other side. It's a push–pull relationship, a give and take, and it acts to protect against sudden contractions.

Most nocturnal leg cramps occur in the large muscles at the back of the calf or in the small muscles of the foot. You can actually produce a cramp in these muscles fairly easily.

Sit on a chair, and rest both feet flat on the floor. Now lift up one heel, so that only the ball of that foot touches the ground. Can you feel the muscle in your calf tighten? Now, try to force your toes into the floor. You will feel the muscle at the back of your calf tighten even more. Be careful; many people can cause a painful contraction or cramp with this simple manoeuvre, and it was tightening of this type that woke Agnes many nights.

When Agnes dreamed she was standing in front of the fire, in bed her leg was probably flexed, with the knee bent and the toes bent up towards the knee. Most people sleep on their sides like this, in the so-called foetal position, with the knees drawn up towards the chest. However, you can't roll over easily in this position because your knees get in the way; Agnes probably tried to roll over by straightening out her leg, pointing her toes as she turned, and this movement probably initiated the cramp.

The muscles at the back of the leg are huge, and if they

begin to contract violently, pain results. The muscle itself has difficulty letting go of its contraction, and so the foot is held in this awkward position. It's an impossible situation, and the impasse can be broken only by passively stretching the muscle. This is exactly what Agnes learned to do by getting out of bed, standing on the floor (making the ankle go back to its usual 90-degree angle) and massaging the cramp.

Remember, nocturnal leg cramps occur in sleep. If you regularly experience cramping in the calf during the day, see your doctor.

ANOTHER CAUSE OF CRAMPS

Another important cause of cramps is irritability of the muscles, usually from overuse, such as excessive exercise, or improper use, which is much more frequent. This cause is common among older people. As we age, the ligaments in the foot and ankle weaken, the arches fall and the anatomy of the foot changes, with the result that the dynamics of weight-bearing alter dramatically. This often means that more strain is put on the muscles of the calf (because they're now pulling at a different angle), and the muscles become more likely to cramp. Proper attention to the dynamics of weight-bearing in the foot, by the use of such things as custom-made supports worn inside your shoes (called 'orthotics'), will often decrease the irritability of the muscles, and thus decrease, or stop, nighttime cramping.

Wearing proper shoes during the day can decrease the strain on these muscles and prevent nighttime cramping. The interest in recreational jogging that has emerged over the past few years has led to improvements in shoe design and a focus on the practical understanding of the biomechanics of the foot. Thus trainers offer by far the best support, cushioning and alignment. Wearing trainers all day may very well help you sleep better all night.

It is true that low calcium, low potassium, low sodium, renal failure and other metabolic abnormalities can produce leg cramping, as can some medicines, but these are rare causes; most patients with leg cramps at night have no demonstrable chemical abnormality or underlying disease.

TIPS FOR SLEEPERS WITH LEG CRAMPS

1. The most common cause of leg cramping at night is a physical tendency of the muscles to shorten. Try to stretch the affected area before retiring. The best single exercise to stretch the calf muscles consists of standing about three feet (a metre) from a wall and then leaning forward to touch the wall with your hands, leaving your heels flat on the floor. You can feel the muscles stretch. Massage and heat also help, as do simple rhythmic exercise routines before bed.

2. Try not to point your toes while lying flat in bed. This sounds silly, but anything that causes you to point your toe predisposes you to have leg cramps. Heavy bedclothes tightly tucked in, sleeping on your stomach, stretching out in bed while turning – all set the stage for severe contraction of the calf muscles. Untuck and lift out the covers at the foot of the bed, or use some kind of cradle at your feet to keep the covers off them, preventing the weight of the covers from pushing your toes down. Turning from side to side means pointing your toes and risking a cramp, so do this carefully. If you must sleep on your stomach, allow your toes to hang over the edge of the bed so the ankle is maintained at a right angle.

3. Try putting a pillow at the foot of the bed beneath the sheets, to shorten your bed and prevent you from

stretching your legs out fully. This works for many people, especially pregnant women, in whom leg cramps at night are very common and who, because of the risk to their unborn infant, are unable to take preventive medicines.

4. If you do get a cramp, you must stretch the muscle to obtain relief, reversing the contraction by standing up on the floor and lengthening the muscle, or by leaning forward in the sitting position and grabbing your toes and pulling them towards your knee. Massage also helps.

5. Wear your shoes to bed. It's not as crazy as it sounds – though it has to be a shoe, not a slipper with an open heel. The heel will stop your ankle from bending and your toes from pointing.

6. Try raising the foot of the bed 9 inches (22 centimetres). This simple manoeuvre helps many people with night cramps, perhaps by making it harder for them to straighten out their legs.

7. Examine your feet, looking for structural imbalances that could cause excessive or improper strain on your calf muscles or the small muscles of your feet. Many people can prevent nocturnal cramping by purchasing shoes with adequate support, or orthotics to correct architectural defects in their feet and relieve chronic strain on the calf muscles. Invest in a pair of good trainers, even if you hate jogging or can barely walk.

8. Use a magnet. Many people obtain relief from nocturnal leg cramping by simply placing an ordinary 3- to 6-inch (7- to 15-centimetre) magnet under the sheet. Though no documented study has been done on the efficiency of magnets, many physicians have reported that their patients have found relief using magnets.

9. Many drugs can cause cramping, including nifedipine,

lithium, salbutamol, diuretics, cimetidine and ranitidine. Leg cramps are also sometimes caused by biochemical abnormalities such as low calcium or low sodium. Although these causes are rare, if your leg cramps are not easily corrected, see your doctor.

10. If all else fails, you may want to try medicines to treat your cramping. Quinine sulphate is commonly prescribed for cramping; its chemical properties relax muscles and relieve pain, and also make the muscles less excitable. It works for about 50 per cent of those with leg cramps, and most patients have either an excellent response (almost total control of cramping) or none at all, usually within a week, and certainly within two weeks. The usual dose is 300 milligrams at night, 200 milligrams for seniors (like many medicines, quinine may be metabolized and eliminated more slowly in seniors). Pregnant women must not take it, and it does have side effects, including buzzing in the ears, headaches, nausea and blurred vision. Quinine often reacts with other medicines such as digitalis preparations, anticoagulants and anticonvulsants, and you must take it every single night, since you don't know when the cramping will occur. Check with your doctor.

Clonazepam, a diazepam derivative, may be useful for nocturnal leg cramps. The dose is 0.5 milligrams to 1 milligram at night, though it might cause sedation the next day.

Restless Leg Syndrome

Years ago, when she was a young adult, Agnes began to notice a peculiar, unpleasant feeling or sensation in her legs that was present only when she happened to be sitting or lying quietly with little or no movement. The feeling wasn't exactly painful, but it was irritating and persistent, and it vanished as soon as she began to use her leg muscles, either by getting up and walking about or by bouncing or jiggling her legs. However, it returned as soon as she rested again.

Her husband was right: she just couldn't sit still. The need to counteract the queer feeling in her legs was too compelling.

This phenomenon of an abnormal leg sensation relieved by movement is known as 'restless leg syndrome'. In this syndrome, the abnormal feeling in the legs is present whenever the muscles are immobile, at any time of the day or night. Of course, one of the quietest times of the day in terms of reduced muscle activity is just before going to sleep – while lying in bed, waiting for sleep to wash over you.

Restless leg syndrome is common, occurring in 5 to 15 per cent of the population. It often begins in early adult life and becomes much more troublesome as one ages. It is very common among pregnant women, affecting up to 30 per cent of them, but usually disappears soon after delivery. There seems to be a genetic predisposition to the problem, as fully one-third of reported cases share the symptoms with a family member.

Though they all agree it is an irritating feeling, patients find it hard to describe the sensation of being 'restless'. Descriptions vary widely, as do the perceptions of the problem. Some report that the irritating feeling is simply a 'tingling' or 'pins and needles'. Others experience a crawling or drawing on the skin. However, most insist that the feeling is below the surface, a deep unpleasant ache in the bones. (One patient described 'insects crawling in the muscles'.) Occasionally, the feeling seems to be one of heaviness or tiredness, sometimes even outright pain. These annoying sensations are usually most pronounced in the calves of the leg, and they are accompanied by an irresistible urge to move. Sometimes patients focus on the movements that relieve the feeling, rather than on the feeling itself, and they describe their legs as being 'convulsive' or 'jumpy' or, as one patient reported to me, 'thumping'. The poor sufferer is unable to keep the leg still, but the feeling of 'restlessness' is immediately relieved with the slightest movement. The sensation becomes progressively worse as the day wears on, so the evening is often spent in some sort of muscle activity – walking, exercise, leg rubbing or simple fidgeting.

Though restless leg syndrome may be caused by nerve damage from a variety of diseases (such as diabetes, vitamin deficiency, anaemia or renal failure), most affected people are otherwise perfectly well. It can be caused by lack of exercise and by some drugs, especially antidepressants, amphetamines, stimulants of the central nervous system such as methylphenidate, and verapamil, a drug used for heart disease and high blood pressure. It can also be caused, or aggravated, by caffeine or alcohol.

Though restless leg syndrome is primarily a daytime problem, the distressing sensations prevent or significantly delay the onset of sleep. Once sleep finally comes, the sensations may awaken the sleeper from a light sleep, but this is not common. However, if he or she is awakened for some other reason, returning to the comfort of sleep may be very difficult. To make matters worse, restless leg syndrome is lifelong. It is totally understandable that severe emotional distress, including both anxiety and depression, is commonly seen as part of the syndrome. One third of cases have a similar history in a family member.

TIPS FOR THE TREATMENT OF RESTLESS LEG SYNDROME

1. It is important to know the particulars of the syndrome. There is no universal treatment, medicine or manoeuvre that will eliminate the problem entirely.

2. Though restless leg syndrome is rarely caused by a disease state or deficiency, if it is impairing your sleep, see your doctor to try to determine whether prescription drugs or medical conditions such as anaemia, renal failure, low folic acid or B_{12} levels, or low calcium are causing your discomfort. In some people, a low level of ferritin (an iron protein complex) in the blood has been associated with restless leg syndrome, even if the person is not anemic. In this situation, iron supplements may help.

3. Decrease, and then eliminate, your intake of caffeine in any form.

4. Massage, stretching and cooling the legs in water sometimes help in decreasing the irritative sensations. They're worth a try.

5. An exercise programme that gradually increases endurance, especially combined with passive stretching, may help.

6. Depression is a common consequence of restless leg syndrome, and if this is a significant problem for you, consult your doctor.

7. Medicines to treat restless leg syndrome include anti-Parkinsonian drugs such as L-dopa; benzodiazepine sedatives; opioid painkillers such as paracetamol codeine; and anticonvulsants.

Remember, restless leg syndrome occurs at rest. If you regularly have pain or tenderness, especially a tightness or cramping in the calf muscles while exercising, see your doctor.

Jerked from Sleep

Have you ever been comfortably resting in bed, just entering twilight-zone sleep, with the feeling of a long, slow, peaceful falling into slumber as you drift off, the world around you fading away gloriously, when suddenly your arms and legs jerk you awake with one horrendous contraction? These body jerks occur only during the early stages of sleep and are quite normal, even though they often force you to sit up in bed and are sometimes accompanied by an exclamation or cry of surprise. Between 60 and 70 per cent of normal subjects describe such episodes of uncontrollable, instantaneous flexing of muscles during the first few minutes of rest. They are often preceded by a feeling of falling, or sometimes a short vivid image or dream. Some people describe a bright flash of light, or a sudden 'hot' feeling or 'flowing' just before the jerk occurs. These sudden muscular spasms occur more frequently after heavy physical work, increased emotional stress and excessive intake of caffeine. The current theory to explain this phenomenon, universally considered to be of no significance whatsoever, goes like this: during the early stages of sleep, you progressively lose awareness of the environment, and your muscles slowly relax. However, occasionally this process does not go smoothly, and there is a glitch. In fact, you have an exaggerated response to some external stimulus. It's like popping the clutch on a standard car – your muscles are out of rhythm, out of gear, and instead of being relaxed and immobile, they are suddenly overstimulated, and a pronounced spasmodic contraction occurs. Though it does disturb your sleep, there is no disease involved; it's simply a variant of normal.

Periodic Limb Movement Disorder: The Race until Dawn

Most people with restless leg syndrome have another sleep disorder, consisting of repetitive kick-like movements, called 'periodic limb movement disorder'.

With restless leg syndrome, the basic problem is an unpleasant sensation originating deep in the legs, and movement of the legs simply controls this irritating feeling. Thus, the movement itself is secondary, not the main problem. However, there is a more common leg movement that disturbs sleep – and most people who have it are completely unaware. This type of movement is called by the pedestrian but descriptive term 'periodic limb movements'. The limbs that the title refers to are usually the legs (though occasionally the arms are involved), and it's called 'periodic' because the movements occur in intermittent episodes, or groups of movements, throughout the night. Unlike restless leg syndrome, periodic limb movement is a nocturnal phenomenon; the muscles of the legs are perfectly normal and behave respectably during the day.

Soon after sleep onset, however, the legs begin to move, or twitch, in a predictable and typical manner. The movement is like a sudden lifting of the big toe and a simultaneous flexing of the knee and ankle – rather like a clumsy type of kick. The movements are caused by sudden contraction of the various muscles of the leg and are beyond the sleeper's control – in fact, the sleeper doesn't even know that they are happening. The twitches or jerks are brief, lasting only about half a second, and occur on a regular, rhythmic basis once every twenty to forty seconds, creating long 'trains' or groups of movements that continue throughout the night, separated by intervals of no movement. The kicking is usually not present in REM sleep, and the frequency and severity of the kicks vary from night to night, with physical and emotional stress worsening the problem.

Although the sleeper is unaware of the regular jerking motion, the movements often disturb sleep, perhaps not awakening the sleeper completely, but increasing the level of awareness enough to prevent entrance into the deep restorative sleep that is so beneficial. Frequently, the sleeper is awakened by the contractions but, because they are so short-lived, has no idea what is causing the repetitive awakenings throughout the night. The sleeper's bed partner, of course, can identify the pattern, as he or she is often repeatedly kicked or hit. Apart from the resulting bruises, there is another tell-tale sign in the morning – the bedclothes look like they have been through the wringer washer, and sometimes are even shredded.

Periodic limb movement is much more common in middle-aged and older people. It is unusual in those under age thirty, and is found in about 30 per cent of those over age fifty and nearly 44 per cent of those over age sixty-five. Because patients are unaware of what woke them up, the main complaint reported is often simply difficulty staying awake during the day – the drowsiness that results from disturbed sleep – rather than any reference to the movements themselves.

Periodic limb movement may be associated with other sleep disorders, particularly sleep apnoea and narcolepsy. What's more distressing is that restless leg syndrome and periodic limb movement disorder often occur together; most people with restless leg syndrome also have periodic limb movement disorder. These people are literally running twenty-four hours a day. During the waking state, the irritating feelings deep in the legs cause them to fidget, bounce and shake their legs, or keep their muscles moving by exercising them. At night, after they get to sleep (made difficult enough with the restless legs), they endure bursts of repetitive muscle contractions and fail to obtain restorative sleep, waking inexplicably time and time again.

Though these movements may rarely be a drug side effect or a symptom of a neurological disorder such as stroke, usually no specific cause is found. It is thought that the regular contraction of leg muscles is similar to other periodic alterations that occur during sleep (that share the twenty- to forty-second rhythm) such as the regular rise and fall of blood pressure and heart rate. These movements may simply be part of that basic rhythm that occurs when the body is released from the higher control centres of the brain.

TIPS FOR SLEEPERS WITH PERIODIC LIMB MOVEMENT DISORDER

1. It is impossible to diagnose this condition conclusively without a sleep study to record the telling sleep pattern. At the sleep laboratory, electric sensors are affixed to your legs to detect the movements, whether or not you suspect you have this disorder, as there is rarely a specific clue that identifies it as disturbing your sleep. Though you may suspect you have it (from daytime sleepiness, recurring awakenings, an observation of your bed partner, and the state of your bedclothes in the morning), the condition cannot be diagnosed without objective testing.

2. Decreasing and then eliminating intake of caffeine can make a difference in some cases.

3. If your periodic limb movement disorder is associated with sleep apnoea, treatment of the latter often improves the former. See your doctor.

4. The same medicines used to treat restless leg syndrome may help with periodic limb movement.

8
The Sleep of Children

The sound of an infant or child crying in the night is particularly evocative. It elicits in us a primal, visceral response, reminding us of our own human frailty.

Sleep is very important for growing children. It is essential to allow them to remain physically healthy, to be able to flourish and grow, and to learn. It's also indispensable for their emotional development, their growing sense of enjoyment and pleasure and their sense of humour.

Unfortunately, even though sleep is so significant, for many growing children regularly achieving adequate sleep is far from straightforward.

As any mother knows, newborn babies sleep much of the time, but their periods of wakefulness have nothing to do with the usual daylight–dark cycle. Older infants also frequently cause sleep difficulties, not so much for themselves, but for the rest of the family. In contrast, young children are usually excellent sleepers; they go to bed when they are tired, sleep fairly soundly and wake up refreshed. Unfortunately, young children also experience disturbing sleep events such as night terrors and sleepwalking. Teenagers have their own sleep problems, the most frequent of which is that they allow extrinsic pressures to reduce their sleep time. No longer responsive to their own inner need for sleep (as are younger children), teenagers imitate adult patterns and begin to allow homework, television and social events to delay and shorten their sleep, and most teenagers are chronically sleep deprived as a result.

Newborns: The Original Sleep Machines

Newborn infants are excellent sleepers, spending about 70 per cent of their time asleep – about sixteen to seventeen of each twenty-four hours. Usually they will sleep for short periods of three to four hours, and then will awaken and remain awake and alert for one to two hours. This short cycling is normal, fairly regular and predictable. However, there is quite a bit of variation in the amount of sleep needed by newborns; some infants need as little as ten to twelve hours, but even these infants demonstrate a short cycle of three and a half to four hours' sleep followed by a period of wakefulness. Fifty to 60 per cent of the sleep of newborns is REM or dream sleep, but it is not associated with profound muscular paralysis as it is in adults; their paralysis is often only partial, and frequently sucking motions, facial grimaces, stretching of arms and legs and even smiling occur during their sleep.

The main sleep problem of newborns is simply that their sleep–wake cycle is not geared to any external clues, like daylight. It seems that a normal sleep–wake pattern (of an older child or adult) depends on two things: further development of the connections within the brain and between the brain and the retina of the eye, and regular exposure to some bright light and dark. Newborns feed and sleep all day and all night long, and the most common sleep disturbance is one they create for others, especially their mothers. Pregnant women don't sleep well, especially during the last few months of pregnancy, and sleep is often markedly disturbed by labour and delivery. After delivery, the excitement that accompanies the event often prevents the mother from re-establishing her own restful sleep, especially if she is in hospital. Mothers

---

Tips to Help Your Newborn Sleep

1. Usually newborn babies sleep very well by themselves. If they don't, consult your doctor to determine whether or not any medical problem, such as colic, infection or allergy, is present.
2. Cow's milk allergy can be very easy to diagnose, and allergy to breast milk does not occur. However, some of the chemicals and foods ingested by the mother may be contaminating the breast milk and causing sleeplessness. Monitor your diet and chemical intake, and consult your doctor.
3. Mothers of newborns should try to adapt their schedule to that of the baby. Caring for a newborn is full-time work, and it helps if you have some assistance with some of your other chores. Take advantage of the time when your infant sleeps – be it only for three hours at a stretch – and expect to sleep more than usual (because your sleep will be fragmented).
4. Never give sleep medications to newborns.

---

must recognize the inherent short sleep–wake cycles of newborns and try to focus on their own sleep pattern, especially to maximize their rest when the infant sleeps.

By age three months, the newborn's brain has matured rapidly to the stage where sleep EEG patterns are essentially the same as those of adults. Most babies at this time begin to consolidate their sleep into one long period at night and spend a larger percentage of time awake during the daylight hours. This is really a period of conditioning during which the daylight and darkness help to establish the maturing sleep–wake cycle. By about three months, REM sleep is no longer the dominant sleep pattern; rather, deep sleep is. By sixteen weeks, the total sleep time also decreases to a level of fourteen or fifteen hours per day, though there is wide variation.

Colic and Allergy: Two Good Reasons Why Your Baby Won't Sleep

Infantile colic consists of regular episodes of inconsolable fussiness. It occurs in one out of every five babies, and very commonly causes disturbed sleep. Typically, the infant seems fine during the day, but late in the afternoon or early evening has episodes of violent, recurring screaming attacks – often lasting for hours. During these attacks, the baby cannot be settled – he or she will pull up the legs as if in cramps, will demonstrate facial grimacing and will actively move the arms and legs, with stiffening and flailing. The episodes quite commonly last more than three hours per day and recur regularly. The cause of colic is not known, but it is thought to be related to a delayed development of the bowel. It spontaneously disappears by about four months. Infantile colic is usually not present at birth, but develops after about ten to fourteen days of life.

In general, infants with colic are very poor sleepers – they have difficulty falling asleep and frequently waken, and they are very sensitive to changes in the sleep–wake cycle and routine. They seem to be much more aware of their external environment than are other infants. Unfortunately, a baby who has colic is more likely to have difficulty sleeping as an infant or older child.

A second common cause for difficulty with sleep in newborns is cow's milk allergy, which occurs in about one in every six infants, and there is a genetic predisposition to it. Classic signs of severe milk allergy include vomiting, profuse diarrhoea, irritability and bloating. When these symptoms occur in an infant fed cow's milk formula soon after birth, the diagnosis is usually easy. However, infants

---

Tips to Help Prevent Sudden Infant Death Syndrome

1. Babies should not be allowed to sleep face down. They should be put to sleep on their back, or on their side (with the lower arm well forward so the infant will not roll forward onto their front).
2. Don't smoke during pregnancy (or any other time, for that matter). Don't smoke around infants or babies – they are entitled to a fair chance at life. If you cannot stop smoking for your own sake, or for the sake of your children, then you must smoke outside.
3. Don't allow your infant to become too warm or too cold. If in doubt, check the baby's temperature or the temperature of the room. This is very important during an upper respiratory infection.
4. Seek medical help if your baby is unwell. Viral infections and fevers may need less, not more, bedding and clothing.

---

who have a milder form may not have vomiting or diarrhoea, but simply bloating and irritability. Of great importance is the concept that a newborn baby with milk allergy may be noted by the parents to be simply irritable – not settling as quickly, perhaps seeming to be in pain, or simply not a happy child. These babies always sleep poorly – they have difficulty getting to sleep and they awaken often.

Treatment is quite straightforward. Try the infant on a formula that does not contain cow's milk protein – for example, a soy-protein based product.

Is Cot Death a Sleep Disorder?

Cot death, or Sudden Infant Death Syndrome (SIDS) is defined as 'a sudden and unexpected death of an infant or young child, in which a thorough postmortem examination, and examination of the death scene, fails to demonstrate an adequate cause for death'. It is the single most frequent cause of infant death, accounting for about 295 deaths a year in the UK and 3,000 deaths a year in the United States.

The stories are basically the same. Usually, a perfectly healthy, happy baby is settled down for a little nap or bedtime without any hint of anything amiss. When the mother goes in to wake up the infant, she finds her child dead – blue and very still. Resuscitation is attempted, the ambulance called and the baby arrives in a hospital casualty department, where doctors try to resurrect the infant. The tiny hope of life that was the baby has been extinguished, and no one knows why.

Three-quarters of the deaths occur in infants between the ages of two and four months, and it is rare after ten months of age. Cot death is commoner in male than in female babies, in smaller babies and premature ones, in infants born to mothers who smoked during their pregnancy, in families where cigarette smoke is found regularly in the home, in the offspring of mothers who are very young. The deaths most often occur during the cold season in temperate climates. One half of the infants had some sort of mild upper respiratory infection prior to death.

Significantly, cot death occurs more frequently when infants are allowed to sleep in a prone or face-down position and when infants are more heavily wrapped. Recent studies at Bristol University also showed that bed sharing with the mother was safer than bed sharing with the father.

Bed sharing with a parent who had taken alcohol was another risk factor and sleeping on a sofa with a parent increased the risks 16 fold. In New Zealand, where cot death rates are inexplicably high, a campaign to educate mothers has resulted in a dramatic decrease in incidence (almost 50 per cent over two years).

Cot death may be a sleep disorder, though the evidence is not conclusive. Most such deaths occur either during the night or during nap time, suggesting a relationship with sleep. Parents who happened to be in the same room with their child at the time of death most often report that no crying was heard, raising the suspicion that the death may have occurred during sleep. We know that the ability to react to low oxygen levels in the blood is reduced during REM sleep, and the percentage of REM sleep is much higher in young infants than it is in older children and adults. We also know that sleep disturbances, including apnoea, are commoner in premature infants (who again have a greater amount of REM sleep). All these observations suggest that cot death may be related to sleep.

When cot death infants are examined carefully at autopsy, the only consistent finding is that of small groupings of fresh bruises – microscopic areas of bleeding – on the lungs and the lining of the heart. Exactly the same pattern is seen in infants who die in choking spells or from obstruction of their upper airway, suggesting that the final mechanism for cot death may be the same.

However, conclusive evidence linking cot death to a sleep disorder is lacking. Much of the clinically observed information doesn't fit this hypothesis, and the suspicion is that the phenomenon is much more complicated than a simple sleep disorder, though it may occur during sleep.

Sleep Problems in Infants and Young Children

By six months of age, most infants sleep thirteen to fourteen hours a day, and most of this occurs in one fairly long, uninterrupted period at night, plus two naps a day, each one to two hours long. Their sleep cycle is basically the same as an adult's. As the brain has developed the percentage of REM sleep has fallen to close to the adult level of 25 per cent of the total sleep time.

Unfortunately, this is often a very difficult time to establish good sleep patterns, and many families regularly experience disrupted sleep for months as infants repeatedly awaken throughout the night and cry out. Most of these infants are perfectly well. Though they awaken frequently and cry lustily throughout the night, the infants themselves are not sleep deprived – they are, of course, allowed to sleep in until their intrinsic sleep need has been satisfied – but the rest of the family becomes irritable and moody, frustrated and guilty. Though the sleep of the infant is disturbed, usually the family suffers more than the child.

Help Your Child Learn to Sleep

Oddly, children are not born with an innate ability to sleep well. Proper, refreshing sleep does not come naturally to all of them; it needs some nurturing, some attention to detail. One of the important tasks of new parents is to teach their offspring how to sleep well.

Just as for Pavlov's dogs, conditioning is often the root of the problem. Look at it from the baby's point of view and this becomes clear. At bedtime, the baby is held or rocked, perhaps sung to, wrapped snugly and fed warm milk. An older infant is placed in a crib or bassinet and rocked or patted until sleep finally comes. Usually going to sleep is not a great difficulty in young infants under one year of age, and sleep comes quickly and fairly easily.

When a toddler wakes up, which normally happens six to eight times each night, he or she is unable to fall back to sleep, and so cries out for help. Why can't the infant fall back to sleep? The answer is simple: the infant has learned to associate many types of sensory stimulation with going to sleep, and none of these is available when the baby wakes up at night. There is no soft voice in the darkened room, there is no soothing coo or soft lullaby, there is no milk to settle with, no physical contact such as a rub or a pat, and without these Pavlovian 'bells' that signal sleep to the infant, it is no wonder that he or she cannot easily drift off to sleep again. The idea that we actually learn to be able to fall asleep very early in life by associating various things in the environment and various sensory stimulations with the process of falling asleep is important. Think of your own presleep rituals and associations, such as brushing your teeth.

Infants must be taught to be able to go to sleep on their own, without a parent present; without being held, rocked, patted or sung to; and without being fed, suckled or given a pacifier. The repeated awakenings, which are quite normal, will persist, but the infant will have learned that he or she is able to fall asleep again without assistance.

Other Common Causes of Cries in the Night

Another common cause of repeated awakenings with crying is overfeeding. If the child is being fed far too much, this causes the crying throughout the night. Too much fluid causes more urine than normal to be produced overnight. This overdistends the bladder, which sends a sensory stimulus to the brain, which may awaken the child. Excessive wetting produces very soggy and heavy diapers (a tell-tale sign in the morning), and the evaporation of this urine may lower this child's skin temperature and cause awakening as well. Overfeeding creates the pangs of hunger – a hunger that is not a natural need for food, but rather is more of a conditioned or learned need for the pattern of feeding that occurs at night. The infant is being taught to associate feeding with going to sleep.

Obviously, this whole process escalates when you feed an infant older than six months of age who awakens at night. You are reinforcing the problem, teaching a pattern of disturbed, segmented sleep, which is counterproductive. The association of food with going back to sleep that you are teaching your child is hard to break.

Treatment is simple – it consists of a very gradual reduction in the amount of feeding before bed, and total elimination of feeding throughout the night. Gradual is the important word here; a marked change over two or three nights will worsen, not improve, the sleep disorder. Most six-month-old infants no longer need a nighttime feeding, and certainly, by eight months of age, there is no nutritional reason for it.

Rhythmic Disorders in Young Children

It is quite disturbing to parents to see their young child perform some kind of rocking or moving when going to sleep, or during early sleep. In fact, these rhythmic events are very common, and usually quite innocent. Unfortunately, they have a bad connotation, as they are also associated with mental retardation, brain injury and other serious medical problems. Most children with these simple rhythmic movements are developmentally, behaviourally and medically quite normal.

Simple body rocking or shuttling is one of the earliest rhythmic patterns to occur, often beginning at about six months of age, and, like all the actions in this group, is usually seen at sleep onset, as the child is settling in the crib or bed, or in the early stages of sleep. It's characterized by a swaying or rocking of the entire body while the child is supported on hands and knees. The activity is often fairly mild, and seems to be pleasurable. It may occur nightly, and lasts fifteen minutes or less. As the child ages, this symptom may progress to the more violent head banging at about nine months of age. This movement is characterized by forceful forwards–backwards movement of the head in a rocking manner, with the head hitting the pillow or mattress, or sometimes even a firmer surface, such as the edge of the crib. Physical injury is quite rare. Doctors are not sure why these movements occur, but it is postulated that it is some sort of stimulation to the balance system that has become a learned habit. The third common rhythmic pattern to appear is head rolling, often seen at about ten to twelve months of age. This pattern involves the child's moving the head (and occasionally the entire body) from one side to the other while lying on his or her back.

These rhythmic movements often disappear spontaneously between ages two and four years, and – this cannot be emphasized too much – are usually *normal* developmental variants. No treatment is necessary, and injury is very rare. When these stereotypical movements persist into older childhood, or when they intrude into wakefulness, they may have an associated emotional conflict, but most instances of this common type of behaviour simply become less frequent and cease as the child ages, leaving no trace behind.

Sleep Apnoea in Childhood

Sleep apnoea is common in children, as well as adults, though the cause is somewhat different. In children, the obstructive mechanism of sleep apnoea is caused by increase in size of the lymphoid tissue of the tonsils and adenoids. In many children, these tissues are large enough to cause obstruction even during the day; they must breathe through their mouth and, during sleep, when the tissues relax, the airway collapses, and a cycle of loud snoring alternating with periods of stoppage of breathing, followed by an awakening, repeats itself. These children usually have excessive daytime sleepiness, and consequently poor school performance, headaches, irritability and a general lack of interest in life.

Much the same kind of obstruction of air flow can be caused by allergies, when the tissues in the nose and the back of the throat become swollen because of inhaled pollen or other allergens.

Treatment of the cause of the obstruction quickly reverses the problem.

The Demons of Childhood: Persisting Fears and Nightmares in Children

Newborns and young infants have no fear, but as a child develops and begins to understand the concept of self and separation from others, the development of some amount of fear is normal; it's part of growing up. Unfortunately, the more unstable the environment, the more likely the child is to have disturbing fears. When a child lies alone in bed at night, it is not surprising that, surrounded by the darkness that incites imagination, fear may overtake him.

Most fears in childhood are transient and easily understood. The world is difficult to explain and comprehend, even for adults, and such things as fire, death within the family, violence of any sort and the bombardment of frightening images that are part of everyday life (thanks to television and films) are obvious sources of transient fears and nightmares. Most of the fear that attends these occurrences can be offset with firm support and explanation. A child who wakes at night after a nightmare, or who cannot get to sleep because of a frightening image, needs reassurance from a parent.

Sometimes, however, fears persist, and occasionally intrude on the waking thoughts of the child. This sort of fear may require professional psychological help if it persists.

All children dream, as they spend a significant portion of time in REM sleep. Premature infants spend most of their resting state in REM sleep (though their brains are not developed enough to 'dream' as older children do). Children's dreams tend to be briefer than adults' and to be about the same kinds of simple daytime activities – benign scenes, such as the schoolroom, the kitchen, the playground – and not at all frightening. However, there is a definite sequencing in children's nightmares.

It's hard to get a child to recount the details of a dream before age three, but at this age children begin to dream about animals and humans, particularly parents and playmates. Nightmares in the very young are unusual. However, between ages five and seven, the dreamer seems to participate more often as the central character in the dream, and small-scale scenarios or plots begin to develop. Both boys and girls dream about adult male strangers, and dreams of being chased or threatened, or being unable to move, are common. Ghosts and supernatural creatures appear, and characters from the television and films waft in and out of the scenes. Many children in this age range have difficulty believing that a dream could be so powerful an experience and so much like waking life. By age eight to eleven years, nightmares occur quite commonly; at least a third of reported dreams are unpleasant, and are often reflections of encounters with frightening material during the daytime. In the early adolescent years, good dreams still predominate, but nightmares are common. There is a perception by age eleven or twelve that the dreams are in fact 'crazy', not reality at all, though they are still sometimes quite frightening.

Though young adolescents are generally poor sleepers, the incidence of nightmares in this age group falls off dramatically.

TIPS FOR DEALING WITH CHILDREN'S NIGHTMARES

1. All children have nightmares, which reflect normal daytime emotional struggles associated with growing up. Having a nightmare or even a short series of nightmares does not mean that your child is psychologically ill or abnormal. In most cases, adults can counteract the fear that a child's nightmare produces with reassurance, comfort in the night, and an assessment of the child's overall emotional state during the day. Younger children need physical comfort – someone in the room, a hug or even permission to snuggle up against you for a while. Older children, who can appreciate fully the difference between the real world and the dream world, need discussion

during the waking hours to explain their dreams.

2. Distinguish between nightmares and night terrors. Nightmares usually occur in the second half of the night, when dreams are most intense. Night terrors usually occur earlier – within one to two hours of falling asleep. During a nightmare, though crying and frightened, the child is usually aware of your presence and responds to it. In contrast, during night terrors the child usually has the appearance of severe fright, anger and confusion, and is not aware of your presence during the episode. After a nightmare, many children have difficulty falling back to sleep because of the persisting fear, but after night terrors the return to sleep is usually rapid. A nightmare may not be forgotten in the morning, but the night terror always is.

3. Frequent or recurring nightmares often reflect more intense psychological stress, instability in the child's life or emotional difficulties. Nightmares are much more common in families undergoing divorce, or where sickness, injury or death has occurred. Any frightening experience increases the number of nightmares. For persistent or severe nightmares, professional counselling, arranged through your doctor or a psychologist, may be of benefit.

4. Children, especially young children, have vivid imaginations and difficulty distinguishing the real world from the dream world, and the real world from the world presented to them on television, in films and books. Especially in television programmes and films, scenes are designed to give maximum visual impact, which often results in maximum imaginative stimulation in young children. Watch the television programmes and films that your child watches, and don't be afraid to restrict viewing, particularly if your child has difficulty with nightmares.

5. With some recurring nightmares, asking the child to talk about the frightening image, perhaps even to draw it on a piece of paper, can be very helpful. This allows the child to tell you the details of the visual image as a focus for discussion. Especially with an older child, this can be very helpful in allowing the youngster to face his or her fears.

6. Sometimes a child can be taught to change a recurring nightmare and to defuse it with a more acceptable ending. If the child has the same dream on many occasions, he or she can be taught that, partway through the chain of events in the dream, the course of the dream can be altered so that the frightening image does not appear. (See the discussion of lucid dreaming in Chapter 10.)

Sleep talking, sleepwalking, tooth grinding and night terrors are seen commonly in children. These topics are dealt with in other sections of this book.

Adolescents: Who, Me, Sleep?

With the onset of puberty, most young people go from being excellent sleepers to having a chronic sleep debt. Children aged ten to twelve have little trouble going to sleep, sleep well throughout the night and awake refreshed. They are not excessively sleepy during the day.

However, teenagers are often chronically sleep deprived; they stay up late, vary their hour of rising considerably throughout the week and often complain of fatigue and irritability. There are several reasons for this deterioration in sleep quality.

First, the sleep–wake cycle of a young person lengthens with puberty. Most teenagers have a sleep–wake cycle of about twenty-five or even twenty-six hours. This means that their natural internal biological rhythm tells them to go to bed later each night, to sleep the same amount of time and thus wake up later each morning. They are more out of synch with the rest of the world than the younger child is.

This lengthening of the sleep–wake cycle is easily observable. Most teenagers have difficulty going to bed when the rest of the house settles down; they prefer to stay up a bit later. Unfortunately, the next morning, when the alarm rings and they are to get ready for school, they feel tired and have difficulty rising. At the end of the school week, on a Friday night, their natural rhythm tells them that they can stay up later – they don't feel like going to bed at ten or eleven, so they stay up until midnight. They sleep their usual length of time, and end up awakening at eight or nine in the morning instead of at seven. This phenomenon is repeated on Saturday night – they may not go to sleep until midnight, or even one o'clock, awakening on Sunday morning at ten or eleven. However, on Monday morning, when they try to wake up at seven o'clock, they are extremely tired.

A second problem with teenagers is that they allow the social pressures of school and friendships to interfere with their normal sleep needs. Most six-year-old children will not stay up to talk on the phone past their bedtime. They simply cannot; neither will their parents let them, nor will their interior biological rhythm. Six-year-olds respond to their internal need for sleep. Sleep for teenagers becomes a disposable commodity; they underestimate its value and postpone it, and become progressively sleep deprived as the school week goes on, and sleep for nine or ten hours on weekend nights. An interesting study was done comparing the number of hours of sleep obtained by teenagers in the 1960s and the number obtained by teenagers at the dawn of the twentieth century. The study revealed that, on average, modern teenagers get an hour to an hour and a half less sleep per night. The external forces (such as school times, television programme times, athletic and social events, etc.) are much more important to the teenager than the internal factors that determine the sleeping schedule of the younger child.

In some teenagers, the sleep–wake cycle gets so out of touch with daylight that it is referred to as a 'sleep phase shift'. These teenagers tend to sleep the same amount as other teenagers – perhaps seven and a half or eight hours a night – but find themselves going to bed progressively later. They might go to bed at eleven o'clock one night, midnight the next, one o'clock the next, and so on. Obviously, going to bed at two o'clock in the morning and awaking at ten is incompatible with family or school life, but they cannot seem to regulate their sleep–wake pattern appropriately. Usually, this sort of sleep disorder is fairly easily solved by advancing the sleep hour (it's much easier to move the hour of retiring forwards rather than backwards) until it moves through the entire night and the next day. For example, if a teenager goes to bed at four o'clock every morning and sleeps until noon, ask him or her to go to bed at five o'clock the next day, then six, then seven. By moving sleeptime forward until the correct time is reached – say, 10:00 p.m. – over several days or weeks, the problem is solved. However, it is most important to maintain the sleep and wake-up time absolutely constant after this, or the cycle will come out of phase quickly again.

Tips for Improving the Sleep of Adolescents

1. Emphasize that sleep is important – that poor sleep, though it can be tolerated for days, produces poor mental activity, poor concentration, irritability, emotional volatility and fatigue. Teenagers don't believe this, but it's true.

2. The more consistent the hour of retiring and the hour of awakening are, the easier it is to sleep. The hour of awakening is more important than the hour of retiring and should not change much, even on weekends. Irregular late nights, sleepovers, all-night parties and other nocturnal social events are very disruptive to most teenagers' sleep cycles.

3. Many teenagers simply do not sleep long enough. Most need eight to nine hours' sleep a night. A teenager who sleeps in every weekend for more than eight or nine hours is probably not getting adequate sleep during the week.

4. Stimulant-containing foods, such as coffee, tea, cola and chocolate, are very common in the diet of teenagers. These should be eliminated in anyone who has difficulty sleeping.

5. Naps should be avoided. They usually reflect sleep deprivation and only encourage the fragmentation of sleep.

6. Regular exercise, performed not immediately before sleep, is necessary for adequate rest. It increases the amount of deep sleep and the restorative ability of this stage of sleep.

9
The Sleep of Elderly People

Many of us spend much of our lives anticipating our aging. We long for the time when we are freed from the regular schedules of work. Much of the daily structure of our lives is predicated on the premise that someday not that far from now, we will achieve that glorious goal of financial independence – free from the fetters of young children, mortgages and bosses. Unfortunately, for many of us, the goal is not as wondrous as it appeared when we were younger. Old age is often a time not of unfettered possibility, but of mounting limitations, physical pain, isolation, loneliness and frustration. It is a time not of independence and joy, but of trips to the doctor, funerals of friends and daily losses.

Sleep Ages Too

We have seen how the sleep of newborns varies drastically from the sleep of young children. However, the sleep of adults remains fairly constant until the early years of aging. With the other changes in the human body – the greying or loss of hair, the gradual decrease in visual acuity and flexibility

– the nature of our ability to sleep changes as well. It happens to both sexes (though women seem to be better sleepers in old age than men) and is responsible for many complaints. More than 50 per cent of those over age sixty-five complain about their sleep, and up to 15 per cent of them regularly take sleeping pills.

There are many changes in sleep as we age, but generally sleep simply gets worse. The need for sleep doesn't seem to decrease much – the average elderly person needs only about half an hour's sleep less than a thirty-year-old – but there is much individual variation, and some elderly people actually need more sleep than they did when they were younger.

Older people's sleep is shorter generally, with early-morning awakening. It seems as if older people are simply less adept at sustaining sleep for the necessary length of time. The total number of neurons in the brain diminishes throughout age by about 20 per cent; CAT (computer axial tomography) scans done on the brains of elderly people show this loss of volume, or atrophy, and this general loss of brain cells is thought to contribute to the inability to sleep well.

A decrease in the amount of deep sleep is gradual but often quite significant. Eventually, if you live long enough, it fails altogether. A forty-year-old gets only one-half as much deep sleep as a twenty-year-old, and most people who are over seventy-five get very little, if any, deep sleep at all. Similarly, REM sleep decreases, though the decrease is not nearly as great as in deep sleep. Sleep ends up being more fragmented, lighter and less refreshing, with significantly more awakenings. Awakenings are common at any age, but the number of awakenings increases with age – sometimes to as many as 150 a night – and the ease with which you go back to sleep diminishes. Thus, the sleep is less efficient.

For these reasons, naps begin to appear during the day, particularly at the time when the circadian rhythm is at its trough, in the late afternoon. Though the total need for sleep has decreased little, the aging brain simply cannot maintain sleep long enough during the night to achieve its needed rest.

Significantly, sleep is lighter and more easily disturbed as we age. Our sensitivity to noise and other sensory stimulation increases, resulting in more awakening; a sound that does not disturb a twenty-five-year-old will often wake a seventy-year-old.

There are other reasons for an increase in sleep troubles in the elderly. Unfortunately, aging is often associated with both psychological and physical illnesses, which are cause for an increase in sleep difficulties. Such problems as depression, anxiety, diabetes, heart disease and arthritis are all more common in the aged.

For all these reasons, the aged demand more sleeping medication. These medicines bring their own problems of rebound and dependence.

Diseases That Keep You Awake

Almost any medical condition, be it acute or chronic, or the treatments used for the condition, may be responsible for sleep disturbance, especially in the elderly.

Quite a common cause for disturbed sleep is the awakening that occurs with a full bladder. In men, this is frequently due to prostatism, the benign swelling of the prostate that impedes drainage from the bladder. The bladder is left partially full even after voiding, so it has less capacity and fills up again faster. The distension of the full bladder awakens the sleeper, and he rises to void. A similar problem occurs in women with chronic inflammation of the bladder. 'Overactive bladder', a condition in which the person feels a need to empty the bladder although it contains only a small amount of urine, causes repeated awakenings and trips to the lavatory. Both sexes suffer from increased urine production from the use of diuretics, or from consumption of caffeine, which has a natural diuretic effect.

A second very common cause for disturbed sleep is pain, particularly resulting from arthritis and other musculoskeletal diseases. Because older people are more sensitive to sensory stimuli than younger sleepers, any ache, cramp or soreness is more likely to disturb their sleep.

Hiatus hernia, a laxity of the lower oesophageal junction to the stomach, is very common in the elderly and allows acid to regurgitate from the stomach up into the lower part of the oesophagus. The stomach itself is used to having acid in it; its lining is protected from the effects of the acid by the secretion of a mucus-like defensive layer. However, the lower oesophagus is not used to having acid in it and, in the recumbent position while asleep, when acid flows up into the lower part of the oesophagus, the sleeper awakes with burning indigestion, often accompanied by a sour-water taste in the mouth, known as 'waterbrash'. A simple cure for this is to elevate the head of the bed on 2- to 4-inch (5- to 10-centimetre) blocks. This uses gravity to prevent the acid from regurgitating up into the oesophagus.

Diabetes mellitus is more common as we age, and frequently disturbs sleep. Elevated blood sugars often cause night sweats and increased urine production. On the other hand, too tight a control of diabetes produces a lowering of blood sugar during the night, causing restlessness, anxiety, shivers and sometimes headaches. If this hypoglycaemia, or low blood sugar, is mild, the result may simply be an awareness of a decline in the quality of sleep.

Heart disease is a common cause of disturbed sleep in the elderly. Chest tightness or pain, as in angina, is disturbing to sleep, but much more common is the difficulty in breathing associated with heart failure that is worsened by lying down. When one is vertical, breathing may be only minimally affected in this condition, but the altered flow of blood throughout the lungs in a person lying flat creates shortness of breath at night. Often the shortness of breath is not severe enough to delay onset of sleep but is bad enough to disturb sleep.

Similarly, asthma or chronic lung disease of any cause is often worse at night. During periods of irregular breathing (such as in REM sleep), or with any snoring or obstruction to air flow, elderly people with chronic lung conditions can rapidly experience a significant decrease in the oxygen in their bloodstream. This eventually causes awakening – often so mild that it is not remembered in the morning – and a frequently interrupted sleep.

Finally, both depression and anxiety are much more common in the elderly, and both are associated with a shallower, more easily disrupted sleep.

Alzheimer's Disease and Sleep

Alzheimer's disease is the most common cause of dementia in the aged, occurring in up to 10 per cent of those over sixty-five in our society. Though it often begins insidiously, with mild symptoms such as memory loss and decreased intellectual functioning, it relentlessly progresses to episodes of confusion and disorientation, and eventually a complete inability to reason, think or to provide self-care.

Sleep changes in Alzheimer's are part of this deterioration, and disruption of sleep is universal. Episodes of nocturnal wandering and confusion are such a common part of Alzheimer's disease that they have been given their own term – 'sundowning'. This term refers to acute episodes of confusion, disorientation and often agitated behaviour occurring at night in patients with Alzheimer's disease, who seem to function fairly well during the daytime. Sundowning is thought to be secondary to loss of the sensory stimuli that occurs at night, or perhaps the inability to differentiate REM-sleep dreams from waking life – as REM sleep is preserved in at least the early stages of Alzheimer's. Sleep problems associated with Alzheimer's disease are very difficult to manage, and at least two-thirds of caregivers cite sleep problems, especially sundowning syndrome, as the reasons a loved one had to be hospitalized.

Eventually, with further loss of brain function, sleep degenerates even more, and most Alzheimer's patients who are institutionalized have only superficial twilight-zone sleep, with a complete disruption of the sleep–wake cycle. Sleep apnoea is a common accompaniment to the other sleep degenerations that occur in dementia.

Understanding the Sleep Changes in Older People

Many of the circadian rhythms are altered in old people. For example, the secretion of cortisol from the adrenal cortex decreases, as does the secretion of growth hormone, testosterone, thyroid hormone and melatonin. Significantly, the pattern of body-temperature change throughout the day is different – the variations are not as marked. This may be associated with the decreased physical activity or simply a physiological phenomenon of aging. Whatever the reason, it shifts the circadian sleep–wake cycle and causes elderly people to want to go to sleep earlier in the evening and wake up earlier in the morning. Similarly, they're much less tolerant of shifts in their circadian phase or disruptions of the sleep–wake cycle than are young people.

Specific Sleep Disorders in the Elderly

Sleep apnoea becomes exceedingly common as we age. Some studies have shown that at age sixty-five, one man in five has the disorder (it's more common in men than women). Sleep apnoea carries with it significant medical risk, particularly of high blood pressure, lowered oxygen supply during the apnoeic episodes and irregular heartbeats. Any of these problems in combination with the use of sedative medicines, or heart or brain disease, can lead to disastrous consequences if not diagnosed. More than 60 per cent of men over age sixty snore, but daytime sleepiness in tandem with unusual or pronounced snoring, especially when associated with hypertension or cessation of breathing, warrants referral to a doctor for examination and assessment.

Restless leg syndrome and periodic limb movement disorder are extremely common in the elderly. The usual manifestation is that of excessive daytime sleepiness resulting from the repeated nighttime episodes of awakening. The sleeper is often not aware of these awakenings, but the bed partner can be a valuable guide to the history of repeated twitchings and movements. The bedclothes are in disarray in the morning. Specific diagnosis depends on overnight monitoring in a sleep laboratory.

REM-sleep behaviour disorder is an unusual but

characteristic problem seen most frequently in men over the age of fifty. In this disorder, for some reason that is poorly understood, the paralysis usually seen in REM-sleep does not occur. Sleepers suddenly arise from the bed and begin acting out their dream, often violently. They thrash about the room, shout or scream out in alarm, and sometimes perform fairly complicated physical acts. However, they are completely asleep and unaware of what they are doing!

To Nap or Not to Nap?

Many older people find it absolutely necessary to supplement their evening sleep with a nap at some other time during the day. It seems that as we age we can no longer sustain sleep longer than six or seven hours. This results in excessive sleepiness during the day and, in the midafternoon, a nap becomes inescapable.

There are other reasons for the tendency for old people to nap in the afternoon. If one is not working, midafternoon tends to be a less active time of the day. In addition, the soporific effect of a heavy lunch reinforces the tendency to be sleepy.

Thus, napping is convenient, and requires little adjustment of schedule. But is it a good thing?

For most old people, the answer is yes – as long as it doesn't interfere with your ability to sleep at night. We know that, as we age, we find it harder to fall asleep and maintain sleep, and the critical test is whether or not the nap interferes with the nighttime sleep. Whereas a college student or young adult who has an afternoon nap often ruins nighttime sleep, an older person who does so often supplements it. There is much individual variation here, and one must make one's own decision – try stopping the nap for a week or two to see if the quality of the evening sleep improves. Winston Churchill napped every day of his adult life, 'exploiting to the full my happy gift of falling almost immediately to sleep. By this means I was able to press a day-and-a-half's work into one.'

Tips for Sleepy Seniors

1. Avoid caffeine, alcohol and nicotine. All interfere with your sleep, making it lighter and more fragmented. Your sensitivity to these drugs increases as you age: the coffee that you could tolerate at age twenty may very well be keeping you awake at age sixty.

2. Keep your sleep–wake schedule rigid. The hour of rising is a much more important factor in maintaining your cycle than the hour of retiring. So, if you do go to bed late, try to rise close to your usual hour anyway.

3. Don't nap excessively. A short nap may be acceptable, and the best time is midafternoon, but some older people find that a short nap worsens their evening sleep. Try going without the nap for two weeks or so to see if the quality of your evening sleep improves.

4. Because the threshold for awakening becomes much lower as you age, pay particular attention to sensory stimuli in your sleeping environment. Adequate protection from noise and light is essential. The temperature should be constant throughout the night. Similarly, your bed partner's repeated turnings, snoring or movements may be keeping you awake. You may sleep better alone. If you sleep with a pet in your room, the animal might very well be disturbing your sleep throughout the night, without you being aware of it. Try having your pet sleep

in a different room for a few nights to see.

5. If you awaken frequently through the night, look for a specific cause. Is your bladder full? Do your joints ache? Do you have trouble breathing or heartburn? Do you feel nauseated or do you cough? If you can focus in on the cause for your awakenings, you can often prevent them with adequate treatment.

6. Regular exercise helps to encourage deep sleep, and also reinforces the circadian sleep–wake cycle. Inactivity or decreased activity disturbs everyone's sleep, young or old. Be careful not to exercise immediately before bedtime.

7. Many elderly people worry about security at night. Is this one of the reasons why you're sleeping poorly? Smoke alarms, tight locks on doors and even burglar alarms may allow you the peace of mind you need to sleep well.

8. A hot bath and a drink of warm milk are remedies you probably learned from your mother. They still work.

9. Are the medicines you take for your medical conditions disturbing your sleep? Common ones include theophylline (present in bronchodilators for lung disease), salbutamol (in inhaled bronchodilators), propranolol or other beta blockers (blood-pressure medicines), steroids (such as prednisone), some antidepressants and some decongestants. Many medicines contain stimulants such as caffeine.

10. Because of the increased incidence of restless leg syndrome, periodic leg movement disorder and sleep apnoea in the elderly, if your sleep does not respond to any of these suggestions, or if you have excessive daytime sleepiness, a history of snoring, or cessation of breathing during sleep, you should be evaluated by your doctor.

Menopause and Sleep

For many women, one of the most disturbing symptoms of the menopause is a marked deterioration in the quality of their sleep. At menopause, fully three-quarters of women complain that they have difficulty falling asleep, they awaken more frequently, they awaken early and cannot get back to sleep or their sleep is simply not as refreshing. Even in the years before menopause (the so-called pre-menopause), sleep complaints are very common – two-thirds of women say they have some trouble sleeping in these years.

One of the commonest causes of disturbed sleep in menopausal women is the 'hot flush', the sudden onset of a sensation of overwhelming heat, and flushing of skin, often accompanied by perspiring. It is important to understand that hot flushes are not simply temperature changes. The hot flush is always preceded by an alerting of the sleeping brain, which rises from the deeper, more restorative stages of sleep to a more superficial level of sleep, and a rise in the heart rate (by about ten beats per minute). The core body temperature rises quickly and the sleeper awakes, perspiring profusely in an attempt to lower body temperature by evaporation. The sleep has been disrupted not only by the temperature change and the perspiring but by the physiological excitation. In addition, the elevated body temperature prevents a rapid return to sleep.

Hot flushes are not restricted to the menopause. In one study, 19 per cent of women aged 44 reported awakening to hot flushes at least once a week.

Some of the other symptoms of menopause – such as poor concentration, irritability and mood disorders – may be related to the decline in the quality and quantity of sleep.

In menopausal women the use of oestrogen (in pill form

or by a patch worn on the skin) improves sleep dramatically. It reduces the time to fall asleep, increases total sleep time, decreases the number of awakenings during sleep and enhances REM sleep. The worse the insomnia, the better the improvement is with oestrogen replacement. The use of progesterone in addition to oestrogen does not seem to make a significant further improvement in sleep quality. Of course, oestrogen in post-menopausal women has many other effects, including an increased risk of breast cancer.

Though there are no published studies, some post-menopausal women have experienced improvement in the quality of their sleep with such herbs as evening primrose oil, black cohosh root, ginseng and red clover.

10
The Science of Dreaming

Dreams are not the stuff of science. Science usually concerns itself with measurement, with those things in life that are finite and quantifiable, and with the application of universal and predictable natural laws that govern the behaviour of the world around us. As mathematician and physicist Lord Kelvin (1824–1907) said, '. . . When you cannot measure [what you are speaking about] . . . your knowledge is of a meagre and unsatisfactory kind . . . you have scarcely . . . advanced to the stage of *science.*'

Dreams are very individual experiences, our own intensely personal impressions of the people and the world around us, and the relationships we have with them; dreams are, by nature, our bare inner thoughts, purely subjective and illusory.

Like such things as poetry and music, dreaming has an element of the artistic, an ability to produce powerful feelings that can be exquisitely pleasing or disturbingly painful. This extra component, this emotional harmonic, does not lend itself easily to objective measurement.

However, dreams have been the subject of some scientific study, which will help us to begin to understand them.

What Is a Dream?

An average adult in normal sleep dreams for about ninety to one hundred minutes spaced through four or five episodes of REM sleep throughout the night. Studies conducted in sleep laboratories tell us that, if we awaken sleepers when they enter REM sleep, 85 per cent of them will be able to provide details of the particular dream sequence that we interrupted. Such studies also tell us that almost everyone dreams almost every night. Obviously, if you don't enter REM sleep all night, you will not dream. Entering REM sleep four or five times in cycles throughout the night is part of the normal adult sleeping pattern – but it is by no means universal.

It is very difficult to define what a dream is, as dreaming is an entirely subjective process. By convention though, we use the word *dream* to describe the typical mental event that occurs during REM sleep and produces complex, organized, perceptual imagery that undergoes some progress or change. A dream is entirely a brain function and, though visual images predominate, is not related specifically to the eyes; interruption of the major nerve pathways to the eyes does not impair the ability to dream.

Some people can never recall having had a dream on awakening and so think it's impossible they could have had one. Yet adults generally wake spontaneously in the morning with the ability to recall a dream about once every four or five days, although this varies tremendously from person to person. Why the blotting out, the poor recall or memory? We simply don't know, but we do know that your chances of recalling a dream increase if you are awakened and made to get up and walk around, or made to sit on the side of the bed and write down the details of the dream, rather than being allowed to drift back to sleep. This is why we recall bad dreams more easily than those that have no emotional component. We awake more fully from a bad dream because of its frightening or disturbing content. We also know that

---

Lucid Dreaming

Have you ever had a dream in which you recognized that you were dreaming? This common phenomenon is called 'lucid dreaming'. It has been suggested that the female brain has a much greater capacity for lucid dreaming than the male.

Lucid dreaming may be of particular benefit to you if you happen to suffer from recurring nightmares. Many of these dreams begin, progress and end the same way. If you are lucid during them, you can change the course of the dream, directing it to a more benign resolution.

One of my patients had a recurring dream that she was saying good-bye to her young child in front of their house. The mother watched the child walk down the driveway towards the road. The child stopped briefly, looked both ways for oncoming traffic, and, seeing none, began to cross the street. Suddenly, out of nowhere, a huge truck could be seen hurtling towards the defenceless child. The mother was filled with horror and fear and woke up screaming. The dream recurred again and again.

The mother was aware when the dream began that she was dreaming, but in this case lucid dreaming seemed only to add to her sense of powerlessness.

On analyzing the dream, we concluded that its most disturbing aspect was the mother's feeling that she could not protect her child. Accordingly, she determined to try to change the course of the dream. The next time the dream began, she took the child's hand and accompanied him to the kerb. When the truck appeared, as always, she was able to protect her child from injury.

This type of dream therapy, involving guided lucid dreaming, can be very useful, especially for those who experience recurring nightmares.

---

the most easily remembered dreams occur towards the end of the sleeping night, when sleep is generally lighter.

Of those awakened from 'deep' sleep, about 50 per cent will relate some sort of image or visual picture that was occurring at the time. These dreams are quite different from the action-packed thrillers of REM sleep; deep-sleep dreams are simpler, with less emotional content, certainly less activity, and they are more like fleeting thoughts or images than true dreams as we understand them.

Thinking in Dreams

It's important to understand that the thinking we do in dreams is different in several basic ways from what we do in real life. In dreams, nothing surprises us; we are much less critical and accept things as they are presented to us. The dream world has many features of a world of complete fantasy. We can be blessed with incredible power, the ability to fly, Herculean strength or other fantastic attributes. Images and scenes often flow from one to the next seamlessly, and past, present and future can appear simultaneously. Rapid changes of scene, even metamorphosis of characters (one character changing into another as we watch), occur quite commonly.

Three Common Plot Patterns of Dreams

1. Passive observational: In this, the most common type of dream plot, the dreamer passively observes events, often with a marked emotional detachment and without being directly involved in them.
2. Progressive sequential: In this, the most helpful type of dream plot, the dreamer engages in some problem solving and reaches what are sometimes creative and imaginative resolutions of a conflict that can be applied to waking life.
3. Unresolved conflict or repetitive traumatic: In this, the most distressing type of dream plot, commonly seen in nightmares, the dreamer revisits a traumatic theme repeatedly without any resolution of the problem or conflict and awakens troubled, shaken and sleepless.

We also often have an unusual emotional distance from dream events. While some dreams elicit a strong emotional response, many seem to elicit little feeling in the dreamer, regardless of how dramatic the dream's content.

As well, our focus in dreams is different from that in waking life. We are able to concentrate exclusively on what is important to the dream and to ignore what is secondary. There are no distractions in the dream world.

The Senses in Dreams

The five senses are represented in dreams, though not equally. Vision, of course, predominates, and it is extremely unusual for someone with normal sight to have a dream that does not involve visual images. Interestingly though, only 75 per cent of our dreams are in colour, one-quarter of them being in black and white. People who are blind from birth and have never seen any visual image have no such images in their dreams: their dreams consist only of other sensations, such as hearing. However, those people who have had normal sight and then lost it continue to dream with visual images for decades afterwards.

Two-thirds of dreams contain sound, with voices being the most common. The voices heard in dreams are usually accurate representations of those heard in waking life. Deaf people are reported to make appropriate sign-language symbols during REM sleep.

Almost 10 per cent of dreams have some kind of sensation of the body in space, such as a feeling of spinning, falling or rolling. These movements are often perceived as being quite unpleasant and associated with some sort of impending physical harm. Only a very small percentage of dreams – about 1 per cent – feature touch, taste or smell. Similarly, the perception of pain within a dream is quite rare, even among those who experience chronic pain during the day-time. Pain in a dream is often anticipated or feared, but rarely actually felt.

Dreams are filled with activity, but it is usually not stren-uous. Talking, looking, listening and slow travelling such as walking or riding in a car are very common. Active phys-ical work is unusual, and here the dream does not reflect waking life. Such common daytime activities as cleaning, manual labour, typing, or other forms of physical work are rarely represented in the dream state. Only 25 per cent of dreams involve moderate or heavy physical activity: the dreamer's energy seems to be directed to observing the action in the dream rather than actually physically participating in it.

When dreams deal with feelings, they are mostly troubled ones and reflect emotions experienced during the waking day. Unpleasant emotions of fear, anger and anxiety are at least twice as common as feelings of success or happiness. The single most common unpleasant experience within a dream is that of falling, and the next most common one is that of being attacked. Other common themes include seeing a loved one or family member in danger or dead; the feeling of flying or floating (with the fear of falling or sinking); being paralyzed or unable to cry out for help in some dan-gerous situation; preparing for or taking an examination; missing a plane, train or appointment; and being seen naked in public. Guilt is a very common feeling in the dreams of people aged twenty-one to thirty-four, and the anxiety regarding death occurs frequently as a dream emotion in those over age sixty-five. Some element of powerlessness is a very common element and this often produces a disturbing feeling of hopelessness on awaking.

Sexual topics are very common themes. Nearly half of the dreams of college students have a sexual aspect, but the sexual encounters are surprisingly nonexplicit. Most commonly, sexual encounters in dreams consist only of superficial contact with the desired other, such as meeting or talking with the person; sharing an activity such as walking or dancing; or simply viewing the person. Often, the interest

Sleep and Dreams in Pregnancy

Sleep is a precious commodity in pregnancy. After the first few weeks, when tiredness and sleepiness predominate, an uninterrupted sleep is rare. Particularly in the third or last trimester, most woman have great difficulty in achieving deep sleep, because of the aches and pains associated with this stage in pregnancy, and the anxiety of the impending delivery and new responsibility that follows.

However, pregnant women make up for it in their dreams. They have many more dreams than nonpregnant women, and these dreams are often rich in detail, imagery and intensity.

Common dream themes and images among pregnant women include small animals (puppies, bunnies or cuddly kittens), thought by some to represent the developing foetus; lizards or tadpole-like creatures, an obvious reference to the developing embryo; their own mothers, and scenes from their past with their mothers active in the role of primary caregiver. Water also seems to be a recurring image – that of floating on it, as if on a boat, or being enveloped in it, swimming through it – all thought to be references to the amniotic fluid, the personal swimming pool that surrounds their developing infant; and architecture – houses, containers, boxes or other shapes symbolically suggestive of the uterus or womb.

Unfortunately, perhaps because pregnancy can be a time of stress, many of the dreams are not pleasant. In some studies done of pregnant women, some 70 per cent remembered disturbing dreams, and at least half of these were nightmares, often concerning hostile or threatening people; natural catastrophes such as fires, earthquakes or floods; or events triggering sadness, such as funerals, illnesses or death. Thus, although some pregnant women dream of the anticipated joy of the arrival of their new child, many seem, at least in their dreams, to be considering the emotional consequences of possible complications in childbirth and childrearing.

that the desired person shows in you in the dream, though not overtly sexual, gives the dreamer a feeling of well-being and happiness. More direct sexual contact, such as kissing, holding hands, hugging or direct touching of sexual organs, is also fairly common in dreams, as is the viewing of the desired person in various states of undress or nude. Interestingly, actual sexual intercourse occurs only rarely in dreams, and no more so in the dreams of men than in those of women.

When Do Dream Events Take Place?

Dreamers are, of course, asleep, but it is possible for them to perceive external stimuli (such as noise or touch) and incorporate them into their dreams. Studies done show that if you spray a fine jet of water on someone who is dreaming, and the sensation produced by the water is not strong enough to wake the dreamer up, the image of water will often be incorporated into the dream itself. On waking, the dreamer will often report that water was part of the dream. The external sensation doesn't change the plot of the dream, but is incorporated as one of the elements in the dream. It's as if the dream has its own purpose, its own flow, that will not be interrupted by mild external stimuli. However, if the external stimulus is more powerful – say, a loud noise – it may be incorporated into the dream and wake the dreamer up. Observation of this phenomenon has given rise to the belief that dreams are instantaneous – that is, that they occur over just a few seconds before you awaken from sleep. A dream often cited to illustrate this theory was reported by French novelist André Maury in 1861.

Maury dreamed that, during the Reign of Terror, he was brought before the French revolutionary tribunal in Paris and condemned to die. Execution was, of course, by guillotine, and in his dream Maury knelt down before the awful machine and the blade fell. He could feel his head actually being severed from his body and rolling away. He woke up terrified, only to find that his bed canopy had fallen down, striking his neck just where the guillotine blade would have. This famous dream led him to conclude that he had fabricated the entire dream sequence in seconds to account for his dramatic awakening.

Thanks to detailed scientific study in the sleep laboratory, we now know that dreams are not instantaneous, but that they reflect the length of REM sleep. During the night, the period of REM sleep lengthens; the last period of REM sleep, just before waking, is quite a bit longer. Dream sequences reported vary in length with the length of REM. Moreover, sleepers awakened during a dream could often correctly tell how long they had been dreaming (as recorded in the sleep laboratory according to the presence of rapid eye movement in the dreamer); thus, it appears that dreams are not instantaneous, but actually take as long to occur in real life as they do in the dream itself.

Can Dreams Tell You the Future?

Scientifically speaking, dreams are not predictive; they cannot prophesy the future. In a study done with pregnant women, only 50 per cent of those who dreamed that they knew the sex of their unborn child were correct – the same proportion as would have guessed correctly. Dreams that seem to be predictive (and there are some) are often simply the product of your mind's exploration of possibilities for the future that you might not entertain in conscious thought –

dire prospects such as the death of your child, or being raped or developing cancer. In waking life, you consider such things improbable, but during sleep, your mind often examines these possibilities quite carefully, especially their emotional content. A friend complains of, say, a sore throat, and your reasonable waking mind knows that the potential for anything serious to happen to your friend is quite small. However, in your dream, you attend your friend's funeral – you see the flowers and the casket, you hear the music and

Sexual Differences in Dreams

In studies done of dreams, differences have appeared when the dreams of women are compared with those of men. Women seem to be able to report dreams more easily than men, and almost twice as many women as men are able to remember dreams in the morning.

In general, women's dreams are more likely to involve emotion and to have fewer characters, more social interaction, and more references to clothing than men's. Women dream more often about family members and babies than men do, and their dreams are less likely to involve aggression and are more likely to involve relationships with other people. Women's dreams are also more likely to feature indoor, familiar settings.

In contrast, men tend to have dreams involving more characters than women do. Weapons, sexual incidents, nudity and episodes of physical aggression figure more often in their dreams. Men dream more about money than women do, and in men's dreams misfortunes befall the dreamer more often than they do other characters; female dreamers, in contrast, do not experience misfortune themselves any more than do the other characters in their dreams. Men's dreams are more likely to have outside settings and to include more unfamiliar characters.

you experience an overwhelming feeling of sadness. Your mind has leapt from the minor disruption of a sore throat to the realization that it could be the first symptom of something much more serious – say, leukaemia or throat cancer. Several weeks later, you learn that in fact your friend has throat cancer and your dream 'has come true'. Your sleeping mind explored the improbability that your waking mind could not consider.

Dreams Become Medicine: Sigmund Freud

In 1900, Sigmund Freud, an Austrian neurologist, was trying to understand the psychological diseases of his patients. He was excited by recent advances in understanding of the neuro-anatomy of the brain and, with this in mind, began to focus on the causes of mental illness. He observed that the behaviour of many of his patients did not make rational sense. They could neither explain why they acted the way they did, nor understand it. Freud reasoned that these mental illnesses occurred not because of problems with logical thought, but because of an abnormality in emotion or feeling.

He believed that the psychological illness that he saw was caused by the presence of a powerful disruptive force or feeling – a frustration or conflict deep in the minds of his patients. This group of disturbing feelings he called 'the unconscious', as he believed that his patients were not aware (i.e., not conscious) of them. He further suggested that this group of feelings was a force so powerful, and so far beyond simple resolution, that it was destructive and unacceptable to the conscious, logical brain and, as a result, was buried deep in the reserves of the mind – buried, but not gone. The effects of these unconscious emotions surfaced in behaviour, because the unresolved conflicts caused feelings or reactions that coloured the patient's interpretation of the world. This, Freud thought, was the key to understanding what were otherwise seemingly irrational and illogical actions and thoughts.

The concept itself is fairly simple: this disruptive, often

negative force from an unresolved problem was itself in conflict with what the person felt was acceptable in terms of feeling and behaviour. The person wanted the deep-seated conflict to go away, but it wouldn't and it exerted its troublesome influence whenever it got the chance.

Freud found it very hard to identify in his patients the exact particulars of these powerful negative forces he believed were buried in the unconscious. It seemed that it was only when the mind was off guard that the unconscious, freed from censorship, was able to bubble to the surface and be recognized. Of course, sleep allowed such relaxation, and Freud believed dreams were 'the royal road to the unconscious', that the details of his patients' dreams were a clue to the underlying soul or psyche. Freud believed that the dreams of his patients allowed a glimpse into the real forces operative deep within them. He reasoned that, if he could understand the particulars of the unconscious in a patient, he could begin to explain the effect that these feelings had on the patient's waking behaviour.

However, even in sleep the conscious mind imposed some control, some censorship over these deep feelings, although not as much as in the waking state. Freud's understanding was that these deep unconscious emotions were so intense and often so negative that they were unacceptable to the conscious mind, even in sleep, because the emotions they evoked would certainly prevent sleep, an essential biological need that must be met. Dreams, then, were the guardian of sleep, and the feelings that welled up in dreams were not direct representations, but rather disguised forms, filled with symbols and hidden truths. In order to fathom the feelings behind the dream, one needed a system for decoding the symbols.

Freud differentiated the manifest content of the dream –

the literal story, activity and images of the dream with its various characters, etc. – from the hidden or latent content – the real meaning of the dream. He observed that the manifest or superficial content of dreams often consisted of day-to-day activities or objects, and he believed that the hidden meaning of these dreams was in fact wish fulfilment, particularly relating to unconscious sexual wishes.

One of Freud's greatest contributions to the understanding of dreams was his focus on the emotional component rather than the visual images of the dream. Freud recognized that dreams do not contain obvious messages, but are filled with metaphors and images, and that many images were very important emotional clues to the underlying unconscious conflict. Freud believed that the most powerful unconscious forces were sexual, so many of the symbols in his system of dream interpretation were related to this aspect of life: swords, umbrellas, sticks and so on represented the penis, while boxes, chests, ovens and so on represented the uterus. Thus, psychoanalysis (literally, 'the analysis of the psyche') was born, and focussed on understanding the psyche by understanding the emotions and symbols in dreams.

Freud also believed that the early childhood years were crucial in developing harmony and stability in the psyche, and any unresolved conflicts in these early years would often surface later in life as neuroses and other types of mental illness. He believed that the personalities of his patients were essentially formed by the age of five, and he suggested that many of his patients' psychiatric problems were related to unresolved childhood conflicts, these conflicts surfacing in symbolic form in their adult dreams.

Dreams Since Freud

Although Freud's pioneering theory of dream interpretation remains instrumental in the study of dreams, most psycho-analysts now feel that the manifest content of the dream (the objects, the people, the action, etc.) is in itself impor-tant – that a dream banana may simply be a banana, without any sexual connotation at all. Also, much less emphasis is now placed on sexual concerns as motivations for dreams; rather, the whole range of human emotional experience – joy, anger, love, disappointment, guilt – may be the primary feelings that colour any particular dream. The dream objects or symbols are now recognized as often being quite specific to the individual dreamer, shaped by his or her experience and life, and the concerns of the dream are often matters of the here and now and not always the smouldering remnants of some unresolved childhood dis-cord or struggle.

More Modern Theories of Dreaming

The next important event in the history of the interpretation of dreams occurred in April 1952, when rapid-eye-move-ment (REM) sleep was discovered. Sleepers' eyes were observed to move rapidly back and forth behind closed lids in association with marked paralysis of the muscles of the rest of the body and an electroencephalogram (EEG) pattern that looked much like that produced during wakefulness. This was indeed a scientific breakthrough, for it gave dreaming some respect in scientific circles. Up until this point, dreams just seemed to occur by chance and with no scien-tific basis. But with the discovery of REM sleep, we could measure dreaming, as it occurred often and predictably. With this discovery, dreams changed overnight to a measurable human physiological function, worthy of scientific study. The REM-sleep breakthrough launched years of study and evaluation which generated several new theories to explain the phenomenon of dreaming.

One of these theories is very scientific indeed: it suggests that dreaming is nothing but meaningless responses in the brain from electrical impulses sent up to the cerebral cortex – the seat of reasoning, memory, learning and intelligence – from the more basic parts of the brain. The neurological study of REM sleep tells us that, during dreaming, the electrical and chemical processes in the brain are different from those that occur during the other stages of sleep. Automatically generated random signals or electrical discharges from the brain stem (the base of the brain) can be measured during dreaming. These bursts of electrical activity originate deep in the base of the brain and send their electrical charge up towards the higher, more developed parts of the brain. Such electrical discharges do not occur in deep sleep or twilight-zone sleep.

One newer theory of dream interpretation suggests that, when these random electrical signals reach the higher parts of the brain, where vision and hearing and the other senses are located, they cause the random production of images, sounds, emotions, perceptions – in fact, the whole constellation of brain images that we know as dreams. Therefore, dreams have no meaning or significance, and no 'interpretation' of them makes sense at all. They are no more than disconnected electrical activity within the cerebral cortex.

Francis Crick, co-discoverer of the elusive helix molecular form of DNA, has a different theory of dreams. He likens the brain to a huge computer that, in order to function effectively, must have some 'down' time to sort and file information – to process it – to put memories in the memory bank. Crick suggests that this time occurs during sleep. We know that different electrical activity occurs during sleep, and Crick attributes this pattern of impulses to what he calls 'reverse learning', a process whereby the brain reinforces interconnections between neurons that are beneficial to the waking brain and eliminates those that are inappropriate.

Making Sense of Your Dreams

How can we possibly begin to make sense of our dreams with so many competing theories of dream interpretation?

Though a dream has a scientific dimension, such as its association with REM sleep, much of it is art, or personal expression. Though certain content and theme elements of your dream may be shared with others, the particulars of the dream events and feelings are yours alone. They usually reflect your waking state, and include events, emotions and anticipations that you carry with you from waking life into sleep. Dreams change significantly in their content and emotional impact when your daytime life changes. When your daily life is stable emotionally, your dreams are likely to be mundane, but when a crisis occurs, such as being in a serious car accident or losing a loved one, the chance of your dreaming about these experiences over the next few nights is very high. Dreams that trigger an emotional response in you are worth examining because the emotion is the important aspect of the dream. The devastation of loss, the feeling of guilt, sadness, fear, anger – these are the clues to understanding those dreams that have meaning. Remember, dreams don't convey information directly; rather, they speak to you through symbols and metaphors, events and situations. It's the passion, the gut response, that is the clue. It isn't necessary to consult large dictionaries of dream symbols; if you focus on your reaction to the symbols, you can often gain a personal insight into the situation or conflict visited in the dream.

Many dreams have no great emotional significance; they simply review the activities of the day and thoughts for the

---

Inventions in the Night

Elias Howe (1819–1867), the American inventor of the modern-day sewing machine, spent years trying to figure out how he could get the sewing needle through the cloth repetitively without turning the needle around. Everything he had tried to solve this problem had been unsuccessful. One night, he had a nightmare in which he dreamed he had been captured by foreign tribesmen and taken before their king, who issued Howe an ultimatum: if he could not produce a machine that would sew within twenty-four hours, the king would sentence Howe to be killed. Unfortunately, even in the dream, Howe couldn't produce the sewing machine within twenty-four hours, and he failed to meet the king's deadline. Howe saw the frenzied mob approaching him, and was terrified as he watched their huge spears rise and fall. Suddenly, he realized that all of the spears had eye-shaped holes in their tips. Howe awakened with the revelation that the needle for his new machine should be threaded at the tip, the sharp pointed end, not in the middle or at the tail, as was usual for ordinary sewing needles. He drew a picture of the spear with the thread coming through the hole in the blade, then rushed to his laboratory. The new sewing machine was completed that day.

---

future. They are frequently full of humour and joy, for these are genuine human emotions as well, and these dreams need little interpretation. The fact that electrical activity occurs in a regular fashion in the brain stem during sleep should not minimize your enjoyment of your dreams or the insight they may offer you. Throughout all of neurology, there is still a quantum leap from the molecular release of chemicals and electrical energy to the thinking, hoping, feeling mind we all have, a leap that cannot as yet be completely understood by science.

Though it may be true, saying that the entire spectacle of nightly dreaming, with all of its evocative images and telling emotional responses, occurs simply because of the random firing of neurons is demeaning, to say the least. It's like saying that Michelangelo painted the ceiling of the Sistine Chapel by holding his paintbrush between his index finger and his thumb. That also may be true, but the leap between the mechanics and the effect is enormous.

It Came to Me in a Dream: Creativity During Sleep

Though we probably don't learn much during sleep, dreams do have a remarkable ability to solve the problems of the day, at least for some people.

Painters and other artists tend to dream about art, plumbers about plumbing, and musicians music, simply because most dreams concern the events of the day, as we have seen.

When a daytime interest or activity becomes overwhelming and all-consuming, it is not surprising that this daytime focus extends itself into the night's mental activity as well. Intense concentration is not restricted to painters or musicians; all sorts of people make a total commitment of energy to a problem at hand.

Many famous writers admit that dreams have been instrumental in their works. Charles Dickens's character Scrooge has a series of three emotionally laden dreams that allow him to change his ways in the classic story of *A Christmas Carol*. Robert Louis Stevenson (1850–1894), the Scottish novelist, discovered when he was quite young that he had wildly imaginative dreams. He could dream complete stories in a single night, and even return to the stories night after night to change their endings! The plots of many of his famous stories were first revealed to him in his dreams. Once, he dreamed a fantastic tale about an evil criminal, pursued by the police, who was able to drastically change his appearance by drinking a magical potion he himself had invented. This dream, of course, formed the basis of *Dr Jekyll and Mr Hyde*.

Music is also often created at night, and the famous Devil's Trill Sonata by the composer Giuseppe Tartini (1692–1770) was first heard in a dream of Tartini's in which the devil took up a violin and played the haunting tune.

Dreams may even help your golf game. In 1964, Jack Nicklaus, the famous professional golfer, was in the middle of an embarrassing slump; he was struggling to shoot a seventy-six, and he took the problem to bed. One night, he dreamed about golf (of course), and in the dream he was able to hit the ball very well, as he had done previously. During the dream, he became aware that his grip on the club wasn't the same one he used in waking life. The next day, he imitated the grip that had been so successful in his dream, and shot a sixty-eight! The next day he shot a sixty-five! The new grip worked like a dream.

Are you inspired by your dreams? Many recognize that the dream offers a unique insight into the problems of daily life. Those with an artistic temperament respect this unique vision and are open to trying to integrate it into the waking state. Ironically, creative or imaginative thinking is one of the first abilities we lose when we don't get enough sleep.

Artistic insight, that ability to see things in a different light, is a fragile commodity, and is stifled by lack of sleep.

Tips for Dreamers

1. Relax and enjoy your dreams. Recognize that you may be unable to interpret or understand every single image or event in the dream. Focus on the emotion that the dream evokes in you, as this is often the clue. If a dream image seems mystifying, try Freud's technique called 'free association'; say or jot down whatever words, thoughts or ideas come to mind when you think about the image.

2. Though dreams are very personal, it's often helpful to tell the dream to someone else. In recounting it, you must turn the dream sequences (the images, the pictures) into words so that the listener can 'see' the dream as you describe it. This process of describing the images in words may be very helpful in interpreting the dream. Also, others can often see patterns in our emotions and experiences that we ourselves cannot.

3. You need REM sleep to dream, and many drugs and chemicals can influence your ability to enter this stage of sleep. L-dopa (used for Parkinson's disease), beta blockers (used for hypertension), alcohol and other drugs affect your ability to enter REM sleep. Many people experience an increase in REM sleep after stopping prescription sleeping pills such as benzodiazepines, which often results in frequent, intensely vivid and disturbing nightmares. See your doctor.

4. We know that dream recall is better if the sleeper is completely awakened. Keep a pen and a pad of paper beside your bed and, when you awaken during the night with a dream, sit up and write down the particulars.

5. If you have a creative problem, try focussing on it just before you fall asleep.

6. Some dreams can be devastating, with emotional consequences that are incapacitating. If you have dreams that bother you, and you cannot understand or change them, see your doctor for counselling.

11
Drugs and Sleep

Any drug that is used to induce sleepiness, to prolong sleep, or in any way to improve it, is referred to as a 'hypnotic', from the Greek *hypnotikos*, 'tending to sleep'. Poor sleep is so common that there are hundreds of hypnotic drugs available. Most of the drugs will work for some people some of the time, particularly those with mild sleep problems.

However, like all drugs, hypnotics have their problems – particularly abuse, interaction with other drugs and side effects.

Many drugs, especially the more potent or toxic ones, can be obtained only when prescribed by a physician. The prescription lists the drug, its exact dosage and how often and how you should take it. Many other drugs, usually those that are less potent and have fewer side effects, can be purchased without a prescription. These 'over the counter' drugs are generally regarded as safe and relatively free of harmful side effects. The directions for their use are printed on the container label. It is in this group of drugs that many people search for help with their sleep.

The Antihistamines

There are more than thirty antihistamines on the market. They are used not only to break up the congestion of a common cold, but also for such diverse problems as motion sickness, nausea and vomiting, allergic reactions (such as hay fever or hives) and poor sleep. To understand how this group of drugs could have such wide application, it is important to understand the nature of histamine.

Histamine is part of the 'first aid kit' the body uses to protect or heal itself. The chemical opens up tiny blood vessels to let more blood flow to an area that needs it, and also lets these tiny vessels leak plasma (a component of blood) into surrounding cells. This causes local inflammation as part of the body's healing process.

However, in those of us who are allergic, the histamine becomes unstable in the presence of the allergic particle, so it is released abnormally. For example, suppose you have hay fever; when grass pollen lands on the mucosa of your nose, it sets off abnormal, excessive release of the histamine stored there, which causes leaking plasma and inflammation. You sneeze and blow, your eyes become itchy, and you're miserable.

DROWSINESS: MARKETING A SIDE EFFECT
Antihistamines diminish the effects of histamine and, like all drugs, have side effects, one of the most prominent being sedation. In several antihistamines this side effect of drowsiness is so severe that it was decided to market the drugs for insomnia.

OVER-THE-COUNTER ANTIHISTAMINES TO HELP SLEEP
The antihistamine diphenhydramine is the sole ingredient in

most over-the-counter sleeping medicines. Other antihistamines, such as promethazine, though usually used for nausea, cause enough sedation to be used as a sleeping aid. They are found in some cough mixtures.

All these drugs are rapidly absorbed from the stomach and gastrointestinal tract, with peak blood concentrations reached within one to two hours, and they are widely distributed throughout the body, allowing rapid onset of their hypnotic effects. These effects end when the drugs are metabolized to inactive compounds and, though there is wide variation, the effects of these drugs generally last six to eight hours. Because these drugs are primarily metabolized in the liver, their effects may be very prolonged in those with liver disease and in the elderly.

SIDE EFFECTS OF ANTIHISTAMINES

Many patients who take these drugs feel tired, groggy, or dizzy the next day, and have poor coordination and a general lassitude or weakness. Some note an inability to concentrate or a 'spaced out' feeling, or blurred or double vision. Surprisingly, instead of being sedated, some people are agitated by the use of antihistamines; they become irritable and sleepless.

Gastrointestinal side effects are common, with decreased appetite, nausea and vomiting, and either diarrhoea or constipation.

Dry mouth, headache and palpitations are also often reported, and, surprisingly, an allergic reaction to the antihistamines themselves is not uncommon.

In elderly people particularly, these drugs may cause difficulty in voiding, or even prevent emptying the bladder altogether. They also can aggravate glaucoma, heart disease or hypertension.

However, one of the most dangerous side effects of anti-histamines is their depressant effect on brain function, which can be increased significantly in interacting with other drugs – including other antihistamines, alcohol, other sedatives or sleeping aids, tranquilizers or any other medicine or drug with sedation as a side effect.

Feeling No Pain: Using Aspirin and Paracetamol to Help You Sleep

The common pain relievers acetylsalicylic acid (aspirin) and acetaminophen (paracetamol) are used by many people as sleep aids.

Aspirin is a mild anti-inflammatory drug with many uses. It is particularly effective in relieving the pain of inflammation, as in arthritis, and also in controlling fever. Though it can cause some sedation, it is generally not a good choice for a nighttime sleeping aid because of its side effects.

Aspirin can cause local irritation in the stomach, which can be severe enough to produce significant bleeding. As well, Aspirin often interacts with other drugs, particularly other anti-inflammatory drugs, increasing the potential for side effects, such as stomach irritation.

Aspirin is rapidly absorbed, with peak values reached in about two hours, and it has a short half life, in the range of two to four hours.

Though it is not by itself a safe agent to help sleep, if it has been prescribed for some other reason (for example, for heart disease), taking it before bed may allow its sedative effect to facilitate the onset of sleep. If pain is the cause of poor-quality sleep (as is the case with arthritis), then Aspirin may be of value in improving the quality of sleep by controlling the inflammation, and thus the pain. However, its sedative effects are not great, and its risk for potential side effects is significant.

TAKE TWO PARACETAMOL AND CALL ME IN THE MORNING

Paracetamol is a painkiller with some sedative effects, and is used by many people to help at sleep onset. It is as effective as Aspirin as a pain reliever, and just as effective in lowering the temperature of a fever, but it has only weak anti-inflammatory properties. Thus if pain is due to inflammation, as it is in arthritis, paracetamol is not nearly as effective in relieving the symptom.

The drug is rapidly absorbed with peak plasma levels in thirty to sixty minutes, and is metabolized by the liver, with a half life of two to three hours.

Though paracetamol is usually very well tolerated in recommended dosages, a rash can occasionally occur. Chronic excessive use can cause liver damage (this is much more common in alcoholics or those with liver disease) and, because it is so readily available, paracetamol is a very common agent of overdose in suicide attempts.

As safe as this agent generally is, its sedative effects are minimal, and it is short-acting. However, it may be helpful in some cases of mild insomnia where the main difficulty is inability to fall asleep quickly. It should not be used regularly, as kidney damage may result.

Natural Hypnotics: Herbal Preparations to Help Sleep

Because concern with poor sleep is a common human problem – it now affects at least one-quarter of the world's population – many naturally occurring substances have been tested to see if they improve the quality of sleep. Often, a particular culture will, through a process of trial and error over centuries, identify a local plant as being useful for sleep, then pass on the knowledge by word of mouth. *The important thing here is that there is no scientific study involved – just a simple trial-and-error process over many years.* Since herbs fall outside the realm of scientific inquiry, they are not classified as drugs and thus are not subject to licensing and regulation.

VALERIAN

The dried root and rootstock of this garden heliotrope (Valeriana officinalis), a common garden plant with pink, red or purple flowers, is well known to be a sedative and hypnotic. Those who have used it report that it improved sleep and, importantly, showed very few side effects. It is extremely popular in Europe, where it is often used for the insomnia that so frequently accompanies old age.

CAMOMILE

Tea made from the dried foliage and flowerheads of the plant genus *chamomilla* is a popular nighttime drink and indeed has been shown to have a mild sedative effect in most people. The daisy-like flowerheads give the tea its characteristic, pleasant taste, and the leaves have some mild anti-inflammatory effects. The plant is easy to grow, and is a hardy perennial.

Though its effect on sleep is fairly mild, this herb appears to have no significant side effects.

LEMON BALM

Another commonly used herbal treatment for insomnia is a tea made from the leaves of the lemon balm plant (*Melissa officinalis*). The plant itself is a hardy perennial, a member of the mint family, and has a similar scent. It's also been called the 'honey plant', and has been used as a general sedative and mild pain reliever. It can be dried and used as a tea, or the leaves may be used fresh in salads or soups. It has the reputation of being particularly helpful for insomnia in children; in the nurseries of Spain, agitated children are sometimes fed a tea made from lemon balm.

VERBENA

Verbena, which is also called 'vervain' or 'lemon verbena', is a showy plant with large purple or red flowers, and with a stronger flavour than lemon balm, but it is reputed to have a similar sedative effect.

OTHER HERBS REPUTED TO HELP SLEEP

Other herbs that may be used to help sleep include fennel, passion flower, rosemary, skullcap, hops, pennyroyal and marjoram. Ground anise and honey in warm milk is a very popular nighttime drink in Germany; the Hopi Indians of the southwestern United States use sand verbena.

Tryptophan: Another Natural Hypnotic

Tryptophan is an amino acid, one of the group of chemical compounds that are essential to human life and metabolism. Without tryptophan, our bodies would be unable to build enough protein, and without protein we could not survive.

Tryptophan is a component in many foods we eat, and the average Westerner consumes between one and three grams a day. The proteins in dairy products are high in tryptophan, as are bananas and turkey.

Clinical trials have proven that tryptophan is effective as a sleeping aid, particularly for the elderly and those taking antidepressants. It shortens the time needed to fall asleep, increases the total time spent asleep, and decreases the number of spontaneous awakenings that may disturb sleep. Unlike other hypnotics (for example, the benzodiazepines), tryptophan does not seem to produce much abnormal change in the sleep cycle, and in fact the only change (and even this one is minor) was to slightly increase the amount of deep sleep. Unfortunately, tryptophan doesn't seem to work for everyone, but it seems to improve the sleep of at least 60 to 70 per cent of those who take it. It has an added benefit: in several studies, it was shown that intermittent use of the drug is as effective as continuous use – that is, the sleep benefits of using tryptophan at night three or four days a week were the same as those derived from using it every night.

Not only is tryptophan helpful as a sleeping aid, but also some people have found it effective in the treatment of depression, particularly when combined with antidepressants. Many such patients have depressed levels of serotonin in their brains; thus, because tryptophan is metabolized into serotonin, it theoretically should help depression.

SIDE EFFECTS OF TRYPTOPHAN

None of the large studies of tryptophan have recorded significant side effects, though occasionally nausea and drowsiness may occur. However, it is recommended that the drug be taken with vitamin B_6 (pyridoxine) to offset the depression that occasionally occurs without this supplement. It should not be taken by patients who have diabetes or scleroderma.

Tryptophan would seem a good alternative to the more powerful hypnotics – it seems to work, has few side effects, can be used intermittently and does not produce much hangover effect. Accordingly, the drug was quite popular in health food stores as a natural alternative to the prescription sleep medications. Unfortunately, in 1989, in New Mexico, in the southern United States, there were reports of a serious toxic effect of tryptophan. Some patients who had taken tryptophan reported to their doctors that they were experiencing marked muscle pain, particularly in their legs and back, and this symptom was often associated with some peripheral damage to nerves, primarily numbness and tingling, and then loss of function of the nerves. Worse than that, reports began to accumulate of inflammation in many tissues of the body, including the lung, the heart and even the brain. Several deaths followed, and tryptophan was thought to be responsible.

It was determined that the patients who had these symptoms had all taken a specific brand of tryptophan, chemically produced, packaged and marketed by a particular company. In the process of producing the drug in sufficient quantity, this manufacturer had introduced a contaminant, another chemical, which was eventually demonstrated to have caused the reactions. Tryptophan itself was declared free of these severe toxic effects but is no longer available in the UK over the counter. It can only be prescribed for severe depression, not as a hypnotic. Some of the benefits of tryptophan can be achieved by a light snack in the evening, including foodstuffs rich in this amino acid.

Prescription Sleeping Drugs

Benzodiazepines

Anxiety, the uncomfortable feeling of dread or apprehension about difficulties that may occur, is an emotion we all share.

Not all anxiety is bad, and although the emotion is rarely pleasant, it can be a considerable psychological force for change for the better.

However, anxiety can be very distressing and, rather than being a positive force for adaptation, can be incapacitating and destructive. Human beings have sought relief from anxiety for ages; one of the oldest drugs known to us is still used for this distress daily – alcohol (discussed later in this chapter).

The search for safe, specific medicines for excessive anxiety led to the discovery of a new group of synthetic drugs, the benzodiazepines (the name is simply a descriptive term for their chemical structure). These drugs soon became the most popular drugs in the history of pharmacology, and are the most common sleeping pills used today. In the early 1960s, the first of these chemicals, chlordiazepoxide (Librium), was released, quickly followed by its most famous cousin, diazepam (Valium). Since then more than 3,000 benzodiazepine compounds have been synthesized, about 120 have been tested for biological activity; worldwide, about 35 are in clinical use. These drugs were originally designed to treat anxiety, and their effect in improving the quality of sleep was simply a byproduct of their anxiety-reducing properties. Because of their efficacy, relative safety and low cost, the benzodiazepines are among the most commonly prescribed drugs in the Western world.

These drugs are generally much safer than barbiturates, the drugs they replaced, particularly because their effects on the brain offer a much greater margin of safety. With the newer benzodiazepines, increasing dosages do not have the same severe depressant effects on neurological function that barbiturates had; increases in the amount of drug in the brain do not produce further slowing of the brain, or depression of the brain's function. Since depressant effects on the neurological systems of the brain can result in coma, or even death, in overdose, the benzodiazepines are a much safer group of drugs than barbiturates. Fatal overdoses of benzodiazepines alone are extremely rare. In combination with other drugs such as alcohol, however, overdoses may be fatal.

PHARMACOLOGY OF THE BENZODIAZEPINES

The benzodiazepines share various common effects in the body, including sedation, a hypnotic effect to improve the quality of sleep, an effect of relieving anxiety, a muscle-relaxant effect, and an antiseizure or anticonvulsion effect. Some have much more of one effect than another, but all of the drugs have some of the effects listed above, at least at some dosage. The benzodiazepines are all thought to work through the same mechanism; they perform a specific inhibitory or dampening chemical action on the neurotransmitters within the brain, effectively slowing the flow of chemical information from one nerve cell in the brain to another.

Anxiety increases the rate of transmission of information between neurons in the brain; thus benzodiazepines, by preventing the rapid bombardment of chemical connections between neurons that is typical of anxiety, can reverse the symptoms of this mental state. In this respect, the drugs function as governors, regulating the speed with which the neurons interact.

BENZODIAZEPINE ABSORPTION AND METABOLISM

Based on their pharmacologic properties of absorption, length of action and elimination, benzodiazepines can be classified into three general subgroups – short-acting, medium-acting and long-acting drugs. All are absorbed fairly rapidly and completely from the stomach and small bowel, though it may take up to several hours for some of them (for example, oxazepam) to reach adequate blood levels. All these drugs are delayed in their absorption by the presence of food in the stomach.

All are distributed rapidly to most tissues of the body, including the brain, where much of their effect is seen. Their effects within the body are terminated by being extensively broken down by various enzyme systems within the liver. These processes are complicated, and often the original compounds are broken down into other compounds that have similar sedative or hypnotic effects. Thus, diazepam, when broken down in the liver, produces, among other compounds, the chemical oxazepam, which in itself has a significant hypnotic effect, and this compound is then further broken down. Oxazepam itself is available as a sleeping pill. Many of these metabolites are long-acting and thus can have prolonged effects. In general, the short-acting group of benzodiazepines are all fairly quickly absorbed and then fairly quickly cleared (or metabolized to other compounds that have little effect). The ideal sleeping pill is one that has a fairly rapid onset (so as to prevent drowsiness in the evening hours before sleep), a duration of effect comparable to a regular night's sleep (six to eight hours), and a cessation of effect that enables the patient to be wide awake in the daytime. Thus, the benzodiazepines most commonly used for their sleep effect are those in the short- and medium-acting groups; these compounds allow sleep to come quickly, prevent repeated awakenings by acting all night long, and then are eliminated in the early part of the morning, leaving the patient awake and unsedated the next morning.

SHORT-ACTING BENZODIAZEPINES

Triazolam is the shortest-acting of this group. It is absorbed rapidly, and has a half life of only two to five hours. Though it is excellent for sleep-onset difficulties, it does not help if you have trouble staying asleep, because it's essentially eliminated from the body before the night's sleep is over.

INTERMEDIATE-ACTING BENZODIAZEPINES

The most common sleeping pills included in this class are such drugs as temazepam, loprazolam and lormetazapam. All are absorbed fairly quickly, and are all distributed quickly. They all are active, either in themselves or in their metabolized forms, for a significant period of time. Temazepam has a half life of ten to twenty hours.

Thus these drugs should be taken on an empty stomach one-half to one hour before retiring, and their effects will last throughout the night and even into the early part of the next day.

LONGER-ACTING BENZODIAZEPINES

Such drugs as diazepam, nitrazepam, flunitrazepam and flurazepam are long-acting; though they are absorbed fairly quickly, their half life is from two to four days. Thus these drugs, though they may provide adequate sleep, have effects that last well into the next day.

EFFECTS ON SLEEP

All the benzodiazepines decrease the time it takes to fall asleep, allowing you to drift off more easily, and they all decrease the number of awakenings and the number of movements overnight. They usually cause an increase in the total time spent asleep; on average, this increase is between twenty and forty minutes per night.

These drugs cause a decrease in the amount of time spent in deep sleep, and significantly increase the amount of time spent in twilight-zone sleep. Their effect on REM sleep varies from one compound to another, but most cause a delay in onset of REM sleep – the first cycle of REM sleep does not occur as quickly in the night – and most cause a total decrease in the amount of time spent in this state overnight. However, the last couple of cycles of sleep during the night include larger than usual amounts of REM sleep. This is significant because one of the side effects of these drugs is the presence of disturbing dreams, usually seen towards the early morning.

In spite of these significant changes to the structure of the sleep cycle, these drugs usually impart a deep and refreshing sleep, particularly in the early stage of their use.

TOLERANCE

As is the case with many drugs, tolerance is a problem with the benzodiazepines and is one of the big limitations of their use. In pharmacology, the term 'tolerance' is used to describe a situation where repeated or continuous use of a drug fails to elicit the same effect. With nightly doses of sleeping pills, your body becomes used to the medicine; in other words, it becomes tolerant of it. This means that the medicine doesn't work as well – that its effect is minimized – with successive doses.

The development of tolerance to the benzodiazepines is very common – almost universal – and is of great significance. With continued usage, these medicines lose their potency, and to obtain the same effect, the dose must be increased.

DEPENDENCE

Dependence is another concept that must be explored with the use of benzodiazepines. Dependence is defined as being an altered physiological state that requires continuous drug use to prevent the appearance of a withdrawal or drug-absence state.

Long-term benzodiazepine use can produce a withdrawal state, and stopping the drug in this situation can cause rebound of the original problem (for example, sleeplessness) as well as symptoms of perspiring, tremors, inability to think clearly, dizziness, light-headedness, decreased appetite and increased dreaming. Dependence on benzodiazepines is a common complication of their use, particularly if the drugs are taken daily over a long time.

SIDE EFFECTS OF BENZODIAZEPINES

The common side effects of benzodiazepines reflect a general deterioration in neurologic functioning and a generalized slowing of thought processes, especially the morning after their use. These effects can be quite subtle – a barely noticeable delay in responding to questions or approaching problems – or they can be quite severe, with marked disorganization of thought processes, frightening loss of memory of preceding events, confusion and complete disorientation. Unfortunately, the ageing brain seems to be much more sensitive to this type of side effect, and overuse of benzodiazepines is the single most common reversible cause of confusion in the elderly.

Similarly, the cumulative effects of muscle relaxation often lead to generalized weakness and poor coordination. In some, particularly the elderly, the residual effects of sleeping pills, especially longer-acting ones, can produce the same deterioration of physical skills (such as driving) as alcohol.

Symptoms of tiredness and fatigue, blurred vision, a mild spinning sensation, decreased hand/eye coordination and poor performance of motor tasks are all common.

Other side effects can include nausea and vomiting and diarrhoea, and more frequent nightmares.

In some people, benzodiazepines can cause the opposite reaction to sedation; in other words, they can cause agitation and aggression, with perspiration and even hallucinations. In rare cases, they have also caused hostility and even rage, with bizarre uninhibited activity including overt paranoia.

These medicines have very important intensifying properties in interaction with alcohol, other sedatives, other sleeping pills, antihistamines, cold medicines, headache tablets or other pain pills and many other medicines, resulting in excessive sedative or mind-numbing effects. Combinations of benzodiazepines with any of these other drugs can produce severe and dangerous alteration in brain function, including confusion, disorientation and oversedation. Combined use of such drugs is not recommended.

Chloral Hydrate: The Original Mickey Finn

Chloral hydrate was first released as a hypnotic in 1869 and is still used occasionally, particularly for institutionalized elderly patients.

It's rapidly absorbed, with peak blood levels reached within an hour, and it is distributed throughout the body. Chloral hydrate does help sleep, producing a decrease in the time needed to drop off to sleep and in the number of awakenings. Because its half life is fairly short (between four and nine hours), it does not normally produce hangover the next morning.

The drug is a direct brain-cell depressant and, as such, can cause confusion, drowsiness and other symptoms of interference with brain function, just as the benzodiazepines can. All these effects are intensified by other sedatives, such as alcohol, antihistamines, tranquilizers, antidepressants and painkillers.

Because the drug is metabolized in the liver and then excreted in the urine, patients with liver or kidney disease should not use it. Also, it is not uncommon for it to cause stomach irritation and skin rash, and it does have an unpleasant taste.

Newer, Non-Benzodiazepine Hypnotics

In the ongoing search for the perfect sleeping pill, three new hypnotics have recently been developed. Although they all have a mechanism of action similar to that of the benzodiazepines, they are shorter-acting and produce a sleep pattern that is closer to normal.

ZOPICLONE

This drug is rapidly absorbed, reaching maximum effect in about an hour, and it is eliminated quickly; its half life is five hours. It shortens the time it takes to fall asleep, and improves the quality of the sleep. Side effects may include a bitter taste (the drug is actually secreted in the saliva), a dry mouth, some early morning confusion and – occasionally – nausea and nightmares.

ZOLPIDEM

This drug is also absorbed and eliminated quickly, with a half life of an hour and a half to three hours. It improves sleep quality by shortening the time it takes to fall asleep, reducing the number of awakenings, and producing a more normal sleep pattern. It can cause early morning confusion, nausea and lightheadedness.

ZALEPLON

This is the newest of the non-benzodiazepine sleeping medicines. It has a very rapid onset, with peak levels in the bloodstream in an hour, and is rapidly eliminated; its half life is only an hour. Virtually all its effects are gone within four hours, so there is very little early morning confusion or drowsiness. Side effects may include headaches and dizziness. Because of its rapid onset and short duration, zaleplon is ideal for people who have trouble getting to sleep, or who awaken during the night and cannot get back to sleep. (The drug can be taken anytime in the night as long as there are at least four hours of remaining sleep time.)

Antidepressants as Sleeping Aids

AMITRIPTYLINE FOR SLEEP

Amitriptyline is one of the most common types of antidepressants used as a sleeping aid, and is one of a group of chemicals referred to as 'tricyclic antidepressants', as the basic chemistry unit has a three-ring molecular core.

The tricyclics are fairly rapidly absorbed, with peak plasma levels obtained in two to four hours after a dose, and they are widely distributed throughout the body. Their specific mechanism of action is unknown, but they will gradually improve the mood of depressed patients, though this effect is typically delayed by two to three weeks. The half life of amitriptyline is about twenty hours, though some other tricyclics have a much longer elimination time. They are all metabolized in the liver and then excreted.

SLEEP EFFECTS OF TRICYCLICS

Tricyclics are usually used as a sleep aid only if the cause of the sleep disturbance has been proven to be depression, or is related to a chronic pain syndrome such as fibromyalgia. In these instances, tricyclics can decrease the number of awakenings throughout the night, increase deep sleep and suppress REM sleep. This suppression of REM sleep is very important, as depressed patients usually experience an increase in the amount of REM sleep and their first episode of REM sleep occurs much earlier in the night than usual. Thus, tricyclics are used to shift the sleep of a depressed patient to a more normal pattern.

SIDE EFFECTS AND INTERACTIONS

Although side effects are not uncommon when tricyclics are used to treat depression, the much smaller doses needed to help improve sleep quality often cause fewer side effects.

Dry mouth, metallic taste, constipation, fine tremor, palpitations and increased heart rate are all possible. The drugs can cause blurred vision, can aggravate glaucoma and can interfere with the ability to pass urine, especially in men with enlarged prostate glands. They can also produce oversedation, with morning hangover, weakness, dizziness and fainting spells. Paradoxically, some patients experience agitation or excitement instead of sedation, and can even become aggressive and confused.

Almost all the tricyclics can cause some weight gain, especially with long-term use, though the mechanism is thought to be that of increased appetite (this side effect can usually be controlled with careful attention to diet).

As with many medications used to help sleep, tricyclics can interact with other drugs, and can have their sedative side effects intensified when taken with alcohol, antihistamines, tranquilizers and other drugs.

Tips for the Use of Sleeping Medicines

1. Try everything else first. Most sleep difficulties do not need chemicals; rather, they need an understanding of the processes and particulars of this natural phenomenon. Many sleep disturbances are a result of sudden, unexpected changes during the daytime – a new job, an upcoming event, a disturbing altercation, etc. – and do not need medicines, but simply time. Such things as proper sleep hygiene, adequate relaxation, biofeedback, the proper physical and mental environment, and reasonable expectations in life are all more specific and less complicated treatments than drugs.

2. Look at your consumption of alcohol and caffeine carefully, for these can cause, and often aggravate, any sleep difficulty.

3. Heavy snoring, apnoea or chronic lung disease can be made worse by the use of any sleeping aid or alcohol. Consult your doctor.

4. Try to determine if there is some medical problem that keeps you from falling asleep or awakens you early. Sleep disturbance requires treatment of the underlying cause – the pain in arthritis, etc. – and not a sleeping pill.

5. Review with your doctor other medicines you may be taking to see if any of them are keeping you awake.

6. If you can't improve your sleep problem without medicines, begin with the mildest drugs available – the

herbal teas and tryptophan. Often the effects of these medicines take several nights to reach their full potential.

7. If these simple medicines do not work, you may need to try something a bit stronger – perhaps the antihistamines. Avoid using any sleep medicine for prolonged periods of time. For many people, the occasional sleepless night is quite acceptable; try an afternoon nap.

8. If milder sleeping aids are not helpful, you must seek medical help to identify the specific cause of your difficulty.

9. Prescription sleeping pills are short-term treatments only and should not be used for more than one month at a time. Tolerance to these medicines develops very quickly; that means that the effect that you wanted from the medicine will soon be gone – and rebound makes it impossible to withdraw from them (stopping their use after an extended period of time produces an increase in insomnia, which then perpetuates the use of the medicine). These drugs should never be used as substitutes for good sleep hygiene, but simply as additional agents when sleep hygiene, exercise, diet, cessation of alcohol and caffeine and adequate relaxation therapy are not enough to allow you to sleep well.

10. Never take any other sort of sedative or tranquilizer with sleeping pills, or indeed any medicine that may have sedation as a side effect. The combination of alcohol and sleeping pills can result in a fatal overdose.

11. Be on the lookout for side effects from your sleeping pills, especially changes in your mood, thinking and personality. Diminished daytime performance and a groggy feeling indicate that you have too much medicine in your system. Repeated nightly doses may produce these

symptoms only after several days or weeks of treatment. Older people need less medicine – usually about half of the adult dosage.

Nonprescription Drugs That Hinder Sleep

Alcohol

Of all the drugs consumed by humans, alcohol is one of the least potent, and chemically one of the simplest, yet its toll of medical and social casualties is staggering. It singlehandedly is the cause of more preventable morbidity and mortality than any other drug, except tobacco.

There is no specific disease or health-related problem that alcohol is designed to treat; rather, alcohol is taken as a social drug, to alleviate the tensions of life, and for this, its sole purpose, it is very effective.

The word *alcohol* is a general chemical one, and the particular alcohol that is present in beer, wine and spirits is properly called 'ethanol', or 'ethyl alcohol'. The drug is not a stimulant, as most people assume, but a sedative – that is, the drug has a quieting effect, depressing consciousness or alertness, lessening excitement and damping down agitation.

FOLLOW THAT MARTINI: THE PHARMACOKINETICS OF ALCOHOL
Alcohol is very rapidly absorbed from the stomach, and the drug can appear in the bloodstream within a few minutes of being swallowed. Though alcohol can be absorbed directly through the thick walls of the stomach, it is absorbed much

more quickly through the thin-walled lining of the small intestine, so anything that holds the alcohol within the stomach slows its absorption, delaying its arrival at the small bowel, where absorption is faster. Thus eating before or during alcohol consumption will delay the drug's arrival in the bloodstream, and thus its effects. When food is consumed before or with alcohol, peak concentration of the drug in the bloodstream may not occur for up to one and a half hours.

Ethanol is rapidly and evenly distributed throughout the body, and easily enters the brain, where it has its main effects. Though a small amount of ingested alcohol is excreted from the body unchanged through the lungs (the basis for the breathalyzer test), and through the kidneys, most of the drug is metabolically converted to acetaldehyde in the liver by a process of oxidation. This process is a fairly constant one, and the alcohol is changed from its active form to this inactive chemical. Most adults are able to oxidize, or effectively chemically destroy, about one ounce of alcohol every three hours.

Though the drug has significant effects on the liver, heart and blood vessels, stomach and gastrointestinal tract as well as many other tissues, the effect on sleep is consistent and predictable, and is the reason why a nightcap has been a traditional sleep aid.

BOOZE OR SNOOZE: YOU CHOOSE

Contrary to popular opinion, alcohol, though it makes you drowsy, does not help sleep; it always worsens it.

You do feel sleepy when you take a drink; the initial sedative effects of alcohol depress your level of consciousness so you feel drowsier, sometimes even dizzy and light-headed – literally dopier. In some, this effect is very pronounced – a single glass of wine puts them to sleep. Because alcohol allows you to fall asleep more quickly and more easily, many people assume it improves sleep, but its immediate benefits at the beginning of sleep are far outweighed by its disruptive effects during the remainder of the night.

In the first part of sleep, deep sleep may actually be deeper with alcohol; turning occurs less frequently and the early cycles of dream or REM sleep are suppressed. However, as the sedative effects begin to wear off, the drug consistently produces a worsening of sleep as the night goes on. More time is spent in twilight-zone sleep, with more awakenings and much more reduced REM sleep than usual. The end result is much poorer sleep overall – less refreshing, interrupted by many more awakenings (though you may not be aware of them), and a total disruption in the normal cycle of healthy sleep.

Alcohol also consistently worsens all breathing problems during sleep – particularly sleep apnoea and snoring, turning mild cases into severe, even life-threatening ones. Many people are aware of this clinical effect, noting that their bed partners snore only after significant alcohol intake, or that their periods of sleep apnoea are much more prolonged and frightening.

Caffeine and Sleep

Caffeine is one of the most ubiquitous drugs we know. Not only is it present in coffee, tea, cocoa, chocolate and cola beverages, but also it is often a component in a wide variety of drugs, including many painkillers, headache tablets and cold medicines.

The basis for the popularity of all these caffeine-containing beverages has been not only their aroma and taste, but also the belief that the drink was a stimulant that would elevate mood, suppress fatigue and increase the capacity for work. These beverages have become extraordinarily popular: three-quarters of the world population now consumes caffeine daily in some form or another.

THE PHARMACOLOGY OF CAFFEINE

Caffeine is readily absorbed and begins to reach all tissues in the body within five minutes of being ingested. More than 99 per cent of an oral dose enters the bloodstream, so it is almost completely absorbed, and peak plasma levels occur in fifteen to forty-five minutes. It is metabolized in the liver, and the half life ranges from 2.5 to 4.4 hours. Patients with liver disease dispose of caffeine slowly, and habitual coffee drinkers may take up to seven days to completely decaffeinate their blood. Interestingly, smokers metabolize caffeine much faster than do nonsmokers, because of increased liver metabolism. There is no day-to-day accumulation of the drug; because of its short half life, caffeine is largely eliminated from the body overnight. This explains the desire that most regular tea or coffee drinkers have for caffeine in the morning.

Though caffeine is present in many medicines, the chief sources in our society are cola, chocolate, cocoa and tea and coffee. Most people are unaware of the amount of caffeine in various beverages. In the UK, most soft drinks with caffeine are colas, and they have a relatively small amount per serving (25 to 30 mg), but some non-cola drinks also contain caffeine.

Chocolate contains caffeine; an average chocolate bar contains 10 to 20 mg. A painkiller such as Anadin, Beechams powders or solpadeine contains 30 to 40 mg per tablet. Tea contains from 10 to 70 mg per cup, depending on how long the tea is allowed to steep – in other words, how strong it is. Cocoa or hot chocolate has between 10 and 40 mg per cup.

A significant source of caffeine in most societies is coffee, but the method of preparing the coffee is an important determinant of its caffeine content. A cup of instant coffee contains about 65 milligrams of caffeine, twice as much as in a cola soft drink. However, the fine grinding and filtering process, practised in almost every corner restaurant nowadays, produces a whopping 150 mg of caffeine per cup – $2^1/_2$ times the quantity in a cup of instant coffee.

Caffeine Content of Beverages and Foods

Item	Milligrams of Caffeine	
	Average	Range
Coffee (5-oz./150-ml cup)		
Brewed, drip method	115	60–180
Brewed, percolator	80	40–170
Instant	65	30–120
Decaffeinated, brewed	3	2–5
Decaffeinated, instant	2	1–5
Tea		
Brewed (5-oz./150-ml cup)	60	25–110
Iced (12-oz./360-ml glass)	70	67–76
Cocoa beverage (5-oz/150-ml cup)	4	2–20
Chocolate milk beverage		
(8 oz./240 ml)	5	2–7
Milk chocolate (1 oz./28 g)	6	1–15
Dark chocolate, semi-sweet		
(1 oz./28 g)	20	5–35

Source: FDA, Food Additive Chemistry Evaluation Branch, based on evaluations of existing literature on caffeine levels.

THE JAVA JIVE: THE EFFECTS OF CAFFEINE

Caffeine causes a general increase in metabolic rate; it increases heart rate, blood pressure, the rate of breathing, and increases muscular activity or temperature or both; it stimulates the secretion of acid from the stomach, and usually acts as a diuretic. In general, its effects are those of a stimulant, increasing alertness and stimulating many body functions.

Most people take their caffeine-containing beverage for its effect on the brain, and it has been proven to decrease fatigue, increase vigilance, and improve motor reaction time and the response to visual and auditory stimuli. It enhances performance at simple intellectual tasks and in physical work that involves endurance, but not fine motor coordination (caffeine-caused tremor can reduce hand steadiness). The speed at which one can tap a switch increases significantly after caffeine ingestion, as does generalized motor activity. It has a stimulating effect on the electroencephalogram, and a prominent effect on mood, producing heightened feelings of alertness; in some people, this alertness progresses to anxiety as caffeine consumption increases.

As is true of all drugs, sensitivity to the effects of caffeine varies from person to person. Many people are able to tolerate fairly large doses of caffeine without any physiological result. Many others, however, feel the effects from even small doses of caffeine, particularly changes in the quality of their sleep.

CAFFEINE'S EFFECT ON SLEEP

There is no question that caffeine delays the onset of sleep, decreases the total amount of time spent asleep, increases the number of spontaneous awakenings and in general significantly worsens sleep quality. These effects are more marked as we age – not only are we more sensitive to the effects as we get older, but also our sleep becomes generally more fragile, more easily affected. This means that a dose of caffeine that you could easily handle when you were twenty might very well be causing you sleepless nights at age fifty.

The effect of caffeine on the sleep of children is similar, and, though children don't often drink coffee, their intake of caffeine from cola drinks, cocoa-containing beverages and chocolate may be significant. A five-year-old child who weighs 50 pounds (22.5 kilograms) and who has had a chocolate bar and a Coca-Cola has consumed about 50 milligrams – close to the dose an adult receives from a cup of instant coffee.

SIDE EFFECTS OF CAFFEINE

As a general stimulant, caffeine can wreak havoc in many body systems. It can aggravate high blood pressure and cause irregular heartbeats. It commonly increases acid secretion in the stomach, causing heartburn and nausea, and in some people it can cause diarrhoea. Small doses (85 to 150 milligrams) can result in a feeling of reduced drowsiness and fatigue, and easier flow of thought. At higher doses, however, or in sensitive people, nervousness, restlessness, insomnia, tremors and tingling in the skin may occur. High doses can cause convulsions in some people. Caffeine can be fatal at a dose of 5 to 10 grams – the quantity of caffeine contained in approximately forty cups of strong coffee.

Caffeine can produce many psychological symptoms. Large studies have shown that there is a direct relationship between the amount of caffeine consumed per day and the incidence of significant episodes of both depression and anxiety. A worsening of anxiety can be produced in almost every person who drinks enough coffee. Symptoms of flushing, headache, dizziness, the feeling that your mind is racing, an inability to concentrate or to work effectively, restlessness and irritability are all side effects of excessive caffeine consumption. The same symptoms can be produced by much smaller doses of coffee in people who are very sensitive to the drug.

Regular use of upward of 350 milligrams of caffeine a day can cause physical dependence on the drug – and this means that interruption of the regular dosage can produce a withdrawal syndrome, comprising irritability, restlessness and a characteristic headache, as well as tiredness. Relief from all of these withdrawal effects is rapid and complete when caffeine is ingested again. Because the drug is fairly short-lived, the changing blood levels of caffeine over twenty-four hours can contribute to feelings of excessive stress, tiredness, headaches, irritability, inability to cope and inability to concentrate.

Nicotine: The Cause of Many Sleepless Nights

The smoking of tobacco products is the undisputed largest preventable cause of death in the developed world. In the UK 12 million adults smoke regularly. They inhale an entire pharmacopoeia of chemicals – at least 4,000 separate compounds are generated by the burning of tobacco, including carbon monoxide, carbon dioxide, ammonia, various ketones, alcohol, volatile sulphur-containing compounds, formaldehyde and a host of polycyclic aromatic hydrocarbons known to be carcinogens. One of these compounds, nicotine, is a powerful stimulant with a significant effect on sleep. The chemical is rapidly absorbed through the lungs or mucous membranes of the mouth and throat and very quickly enters the bloodstream – it reaches the brain eight seconds after inhalation. Nicotine directly stimulates the heart, the brain, the gastrointestinal tract and the adrenal glands. It causes an alerting or awakening pattern in the electro-encephalogram, an increase in heart rate and blood pressure, an increase in hand tremor, a decrease in hunger and a pleasant feeling of stimulation (at least in those used to the drug), a reduction of aggression and a decrease in body weight (thought to be from stimulation of cell metabolism), with smokers weighing an average of 5 to 10 pounds (2 to 4.5 kilograms) less than nonsmokers. Nicotine also causes an increased facilitation for memory. Forty to sixty milligrams (the equivalent of all the nicotine in four to six cigarettes) can be fatal.

Nicotine does not last long in the body; its half life is two to three hours, and once it is metabolized in the liver it has few effects. It seems that the half life of nicotine is much shorter in smokers than in nonsmokers (they have become used to handling the chemical).

NICOTINE AND SLEEP

Nicotine is a direct brain stimulant, causing increased alertness, difficulty falling asleep, frequent awakenings, shortening of the total time spent asleep and, in general, producing a lighter, less refreshing sleep. In excessive doses, nicotine can stimulate the central nervous system so severely as to cause headaches, nausea, confusion and even seizures. Insomnia is one of the most common complaints of smokers.

The effects of nicotine – indeed of all the chemicals released by the burning of tobacco – are not limited to the smoker, but also extend to those in the vicinity who are forced to inhale some of the byproducts of combustion. Thus, the nicotine levels of spouses of smokers are often significantly elevated. Inhaling the contaminants in the air, including such stimulants as nicotine, is known to expose innocent bystanders to the health consequences of smoking, and passively inhaled nicotine could contribute to their sleep difficulties.

Glossary

Antihistamines: Chemicals designed to counteract the effect of histamine – they are used for treating allergic symptoms and nausea, and as sleeping aids.

Anxiety: An intense state of uneasiness or apprehension about what may happen in the future.

Apnoea: Cessation of breathing.

Bronchodilator: Any of a group of drugs used in the treatment of asthma and other lung conditions, whose effect is to open or dilate narrowed airways.

Bruxism: The pattern of teeth grinding at night.

Carpal Tunnel Syndrome: A pattern of numbness in the hand, often accompanied by some pain in the hand and wrist area, caused by pressure on the median nerve as it travels through a narrow anatomical space, or tunnel, in the wrist. A common cause of numbness in the hand and wrist at night.

Cataplexy: The condition of loss of muscle power often in response to strong emotion, seen in the sleep disorder narcolepsy.

Cerebral Cortex: The outer part of the cerebrum, or higher brain; the site of most of the more complex brain function such as speech, vision, thought, etc.

Circadian Rhythm: Any of the cycles or rhythms in biology whose timing is approximately twenty-four hours – such as the sleep–wake cycle.

Cortisol: A hormone secreted by the adrenal gland; known as the hormone of stress, it has powerful anti-inflammatory and reparative functions.

Deep Sleep: Stages III and IV of sleep (as identified by electroencephalogram tracings), also known as restorative sleep. The sleep where an external stimulus is least likely to awaken you; the most refreshing sleep.

Depression: A psychological state of prolonged sadness, sense of worthlessness and lack of enjoyment, usually accompanied by weight change and sleep disruption.

Electroencephalogram (EEG): The recording of electrical activity of the brain, as measured by tiny electrode sensors taped onto the scalp.

Fibromyalgia: One of the rheumatic diseases characterized by marked muscle and ligament pain, sleep disorder and fatigue.

Half Life: the time it takes for half a drug dose to be eliminated from the body. This is related to (but not identical to) the time it takes before the drug is only half as effective.

Histamine: A chemical whose action consists of inflammatory responses such as increased blood flow and leakage of fluid from capillaries. Found in most tissues of the body, histamine is released in excess amounts in allergic states.

Hypnic Jerks: The common phenomenon of a sudden, marked contraction of several large muscles early in sleep – the contraction causes a single jerking motion, which usually awakens the sleeper.

Hypnotics: Drugs that are used to improve sleep.

Infantile Colic: Recurring bouts of pain in an otherwise healthy child less than six months of age, often accompanied by drawing up of the legs, facial grimacing, shaking of arms and legs and loud crying, and often occurring at the same time of day for several weeks or months.

Insomnia: A condition in which sleep is not adequate, of poor quality, not sufficient in duration or otherwise not refreshing.

Latent Dream Content: In Freud's dream interpretation theory the hidden meaning of symbols in dreams.

Malocclusion: Poor alignment of the upper and lower jaws so that dental surfaces do not properly mesh.

Manifest Dream Content: In Freud's dream interpretation theory, the literal meaning of the symbols in dreams.

Melatonin: A hormone secreted by the pineal gland; its chief function is to chemically alert the cells of the body to the absence of light.

Microsleeps: In sleep deprivation, very short (one to two seconds) episodes of sleep that intrude on the waking state, often without any awareness.

Mucosa: In anatomy, a membrane lined with glands that secrete mucus; an example of a mucosal surface is the lining of the mouth.

Narcolepsy: A neurological condition of frequent and uncontrollable desire for sleep, hallucinations and intermittent episodes of full or partial paralysis.

Neurone: A single nerve cell. The basic cellular unit of the brain.

Neurotransmitter: Any of a group of chemicals that transmit information from one nerve cell to another; the chemical connection between cells of the brain and the nervous system.

Night Terror: An episode of sudden partial awakening, most often seen in children, characteristically beginning with a scream, and consisting of periods of intense fear or panic without memory of the event in the morning.

Periodic Limb Movement Disorder: Disruptive twitching movements of the limbs (usually the legs) that occur repeatedly during the night and often prevent adequate rest.

REM Sleep (Rapid Eye Movement Sleep): That stage of

sleep characterized by rapid flitting movements of the eyes behind closed lids; dream sleep.

Restless Leg Syndrome: Unpleasant sensations in the legs that are felt only when the limbs are motionless, and that disappear with movement.

Saturday Night Palsy: A paralysis of the radial nerve, resulting from prolonged pressure on this nerve in the underarm region and causing inability to extend the wrist.

Sleep Apnoea: Cessation of breathing that occurs during sleep. Usually due to obstruction of the airway, it can also be due to inability of the brain to initiate respiration.

Sleep Cycle: The usual pattern of arrangement of the stages of sleep in a normal person. The usual sleep cycle begins with Stage I and II sleep, followed by deep sleep, then a return to Stage I and II, then REM sleep, then Stage I and II sleep.

Sleep Inertia: A confused or muddleheaded feeling observed on awakening from deep sleep.

Sleep Paralysis: The disturbing sensation of being awake, but unable to move. Though it can occur in normal people, it is much more common in the sleep disorder narcolepsy.

Sleep Talking: Any speaking during sleep – it may be complete sentences but more often only phrases or single words.

Sleep–Wake Cycle: The twenty-four-hour cycle of alternating sleep and wakefulness – the usual is to sleep for seven and a half to eight hours, and be awake for sixteen or sixteen and a half hours.

Sleepwalking: Any complex physical action, such as walking, that occurs with the sleeper only partially awake and in a trance-like state.

Somnambulism: Same as sleepwalking.

Stage I Sleep: The very earliest and lightest sleep, with its own characteristic electroencephalographic pattern.

Stage II Sleep: A slightly deeper stage of sleep than Stage I, with its own specific electroencephalographic pattern.

Stages III and IV Sleep: The deepest stages of sleep, characterized by slow synchronous electrical patterns on electroen-cephalogram; restorative sleep, deep sleep.

Sundowning: A term used to describe the deterioration of behaviour and onset of confusion in patients with Alzheimer's disease (and other dementias) that occur at night.

Temporomandibular Joint: Anatomically, the point in the cheek area where the lower jaw or mandible joins the face; the joint is located just in front of the ears and easily felt as the mouth is opened and closed.

Thyroid Hormone: The principal hormone produced in the thyroid gland; it functions as the basic chemical governor of many body functions such as weight, energy level, heart rate, etc.

Tricyclic Antidepressants: That group of medicines used to treat depression whose chemical structure consists of three chemical rings (or cycles) joined together.

Twilight Zone Sleep: Light sleep – Stage I or II sleep. Sleep from which one can be easily aroused.

Ulnar Palsy: Paralysis of the ulnar nerve, one of the nerves of the forearm, from pressure on the nerve at the back of the elbow. Characteristically this produces numbness and tingling down the little and ring fingers.

Uvula: The fingertip-like projection of flabby tissue hanging from the soft palate at the back of the mouth.

***Zeitgeber*s:** Environmental clues that help establish the circadian sleep–wake cycle – light is the most important *Zeitgeber* for humans.

Table of Drug Names

Generic name	Some common brands	Drug type
Paracetamol	Calpol	painkiller
Paracetamol with codeine	Co-codamol, Tylex	painkiller
Acetylsalicylic acid (ASA)	Aspirin	painkiller anti-inflammatory
Amitriptyline	Lentizol	antidepressant
Chlordiazepoxide	Librium	benzodiazepine
Clomipramine	Anafranil	antidepressant
Clorazepate	Tranxene	BZD
Diazepam	Valium	benzodiazepine
Diphenhydramine	Dozol	antihistamine
Flunitrazepam	Rohypnol	benzodiazepine
Flurazepam	Dalmane	benzodiazepine
Imipramine	Tofranil	antidepressant
L-dopa	Sinemet	anti-Parkinsonian
Loprazolam	Dormonoct	benzodiazepine
Lorazepam	Ativan	benzodiazepine
Lormetazapam		benzodiazepine
Mazindol		stimulant

Meclozine	Sea Legs	antihistamine
Methylphenidate	Ritalin	stimulant
Midazolam	Hypnovel (injectable)	benzodiazepine
Modafinil	Provigil	stimulant
Nitrazepam	Mogadon	benzodiazepine
Oxazepam		benzodiazepine
Temazepam		benzodiazepine
Zaleplon	Sonata	hypnotic
Zolpidem	Stilnoct	hypnotic
Zopiclone	Zimovane	hypnotic

Further Resources

Organizations

British Sleep Society
PO Box 247
Huntingdon, PE28 3UZ
www.british-sleep-society.org.uk

Ekbom Support Group
18 Rodbridge Drive
Thorpe Bay
Essex, SS1 3DF

British Snoring and Sleep Apnoea Association Limited
2nd Floor Suite
52 Albert Road
North Reigate
Surrey, RH2 9EL
www.britishsnoring.demon.co.uk

The British Sleep Foundation
10 Cabot Square
Canary Wharf
London, EH14 4QB
www.britishsleepfoundation.org.uk

Narcolepsy Association UK
Craven House
1st Floor
121 Kingsway
London, WC2B 6PA
www.narcolepsy.org.uk

Books
Coren, Stanley. *Sleep Thieves*. New York: Free Press, 1996. An enjoyable, informative book about the things that rob us of sleep.

Dement, William. *The Promise of Sleep*. London: Pan, 2001. Written by a pioneer in sleep medicine, this book emphasizes the connection between sleep, health and happiness.

Dotto, Lydia. *Asleep in the Fast Lane*. Toronto: Stoddart, 1990. A very comprehensive review of chronic sleep deprivation.

Ferber, Richard. *Solve Your Child's Sleep Problems*. London: Dorling Kindersley, 1986. The classic resource for children's sleep difficulties.

Hauri, Peter, and Shirley Linde. *No More Sleepless Nights*. New York: John Wiley and Sons, 1990. An excellent resource book, emphasizing a safe, drug-free programme.

Lamberg, Lynne. *Body Rhythms, Chronobiology, and Peak Performance*. New York: William Morrow, 1994. A detailed discussion of our internal clocks.

Index